POSITIVE BODIES

LOVING THE SKIN YOU'RE IN

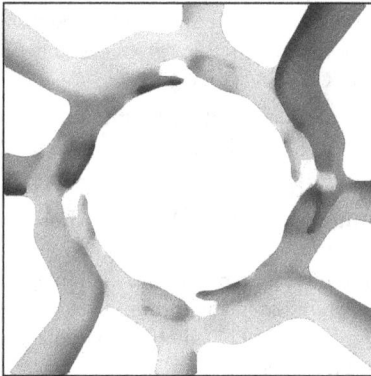

Dr Vivienne Lewis — Psychologist

AUSTRALIANACADEMIC**PRESS**

This book is dedicated to all those suffering in silence from body image issues and disturbances and those battling eating disorders.

Thank you to all my clients, who through their strength and determination to live healthier and happier lives, have motivated me to write this book.

Vivienne

Contents

Contents (cont.)

Chapter 1

Welcome to the start of a positive body image

I'm not typical. I'm not an adolescent and I'm not female. I am 45 and a man and I had an eating disorder. I hated the fat on my body despite whittling down to an extremely low body weight where I was considered severely underweight. I spent all day every day thinking about food, weight, exercise and I was miserable. I could see no way out. It took a lot of work on my part and on the part of my doctors and psychologist to help me see that there was a way out of my misery, that I was valuable and that I didn't have to live with the chains of my eating disorder. I learnt to think of myself as more than just a body. I learnt that I could be happy doing things other than exercise and dieting — that my body is a temple and needs to be treated with respect.

Welcome to the start of a positive body image. This book is designed to equip you with the skills, knowledge, and thinking styles to foster a positive body image. Body image is how people think and feel toward their body, as well as perceptions of the body and the behaviours that occur as a result of this. This ranges from a very positive body image where a person loves the skin they're in to a very negative body image where a person is disgusted by their body and sees it adversely. We know that a negative body image affects how people feel about themselves in general, because our bodies are a significant part of who we are. A negative body image can lead some people to adopt dangerous eating and exercising habits and sometimes dissatisfaction with the body becomes generalised to dissatisfaction with oneself as a whole.

A little bit about the author

As a psychologist I have worked with many women, men, children, adolescents and older adults struggling with body image worries and concerns. For many, these concerns have led them to feel much anxiety and depression as well as destructive eating, dieting and exercising habits that have compounded the problem. What I have found works with my clients is the approach called Cognitive Behavioural Therapy (CBT) where we work on changing the way a person feels, thinks and behaves towards their body. This is the approach of this book. Throughout you'll find examples from people I have seen who have struggled but won their war against body image dissatisfaction and self-hatred.

Body image concerns

If you are reading this book because you believe that improvements could be made to the way that you think and feel about your body, then you are not alone. Australian and international research on Western cultures suggests that 60% of women and 30–40% of men are dissatisfied with some part of their bodies. In fact, for women, body dissatisfaction is seen as the norm, whether this be dissatisfaction with particular parts or with the body as a whole. We also know that for Australian youth aged 14 to 25 years old, body image is their number one concern, seen as more important than family, friends and school. Typical concerns about the body centre around weight and shape for women, with the hips, stomach, buttocks and thighs generally being the most disliked parts. For men, concern with the muscularity of their upper body as well as overall body fat and the desire to be lean are most common. But body image is not just about shape and size; it is also about parts of the body and our appearance such as the colour of our eyes, hair, nails, and skin. Some people can therefore experience a strong dislike for particular parts and become distressed and anxious about their skin, or hairline, the size of their breasts for women or the look of their genitalia for example. A strong dislike for a particular part of the body or our appearance can for some people lead to obsessive thinking about the body part to the point where they are consumed by thoughts of its often perceived (as opposed to objectively real) defect. This can be very distressing and lead the person to spend many hours looking in the mirror or trying to change the perceived defect, often to the detriment of their mental health. An extreme form of appearance concern is called Body Dysmorphic Disorder where a person is consumed by their appearance and trying to 'fix' the 'defect' they see. I have seen people who are deeply distressed by the shape of their nose or the closeness of their eyes, to the point where they spend hours checking and re-checking these areas for their perceived defects.

How to use this book

Feeling and thinking negatively about our bodies can have a dramatic influence on our lives and can affect such things as our self-esteem, gender identity, levels of anxiety, how and when we socialise, our mood, level of sexual fulfilment and eating patterns. This book is designed to help men and women of any age including adolescents and children, as well as to assist parents, teachers and counsellors wanting to help others with body dissatisfaction and disturbance. There is a chapter specifically dedicated to adults helping children develop positive body image. It's important for both boys and girls to have positive body image role models. We often neglect the importance of a positive body image for boys but it can be just as important for boys as they are affected by teasing and appearance bullying just like girls. As well, boys can engage in dieting and exercising for weight loss and become unhappy because they feel their body does not match idealised images of what they 'should' look like, particularly before they hit puberty where they look much more feminine and less muscular than their adolescent peers. For teachers, parents and carers of children wanting to promote a positive body image in children, the first step to be a good role model yourself. Use this book to ensure you have a positive body image first and engage in behaviours that convey this to others such as children who closely monitor adult behaviour. Then turn to the specialised chapter on how to help children develop a positive body image. As well, the chapter on eating disorders and recognising early warning signs may be of particular use for adults looking out for signs of serious health conditions related to body image. The appendices contain all the work sheets to help you go through the activities yourself and with your children including adolescents.

This book is particularly relevant for men who rarely seek help for body image concerns let alone talk about it with others. Body image is often seen as a women's issue or something that only affects the young. This is not true — body image effects people at all ages and both genders. Forty-five per cent of Western men are unhappy with their bodies and one in 10 people with Anorexia Nervosa are male. Men, take as much as you can from this book so you're not carrying the burden of living with body image concerns in secret. It can be particularly difficult for men suffering from body image issues as it can be seen as 'sissy' or 'girlie' to talk about it. The common concerns that men have include their weight as well as with areas stereotypically considered masculine such as upper body strength and muscularity. Men can also be worried about hairloss and the size and shape of their genitalia. You may have noticed over time that the concerns you have with your body have changed with age and circumstance. Reaching out for help is just as important for men as it is for women.

A negative body image can stop us enjoying life. The good news is that there are things we can do to change the way we think and feel about our bodies, leading us towards a more positive body image. You've taken the first step in doing this.

Improving your body image involves educating yourself about where your perceptions come from and changing the way you think about your body and how you behave towards it. It also involves stopping treating your body badly through punishing diets, excessive exercise and misuse of body change agents such as weight-loss pills. How many of us punish our bodies and ourselves unfairly such as going through gruelling exercise when our bodies need a rest, or starving ourselves because we want to change our weight, or miss out on doing something social because we don't like the way our body looks. Body image is just one part of who you are and this book is going to help you get the most out of your body and feel more positive about it and yourself in general. Using sound psychological theory and research, this book is an easy guide to loving the skin you're in!

This book focuses on what psychologists call a cognitive behavioural therapeutic (CBT) approach to improving body image and general health and wellbeing. This means you'll learn how to change your behaviour and your thinking processes in order to feel better and behave in ways that are more healthy and helpful to your overall wellbeing. This book covers the following areas which have been shown through Australian and international research to be fundamental in promoting a positive body image:

- understanding what body image is and what influences its development
- knowing how to change our behaviour and our thinking to feel more positive about our body and self
- recognising warning signs of negative health and mental health consequences such as eating disorders
- being a positive role model to children
- how to manage stress, anxiety and depression
- how to boost your self-esteem
- where to go to get additional help.

Within this book you'll read about the research on body image, be encouraged to think about issues of relevance to women and men, and learn techniques for improving your body image. There are tips throughout as to how to practice these techniques, as it is through this practice in challenging your behaviours and thinking that will lead to better results and lasting change. Scattered through the book are also some helpful activities for readers to try. At the end of the book are the appendices which include all the handouts and worksheets referred to in each chapter as well as references to further research on body image and eating disorders.

It is expected that this book will help increase your body and life satisfaction and reduce body distress and anxiety through doing the activities suggested. It will increase your awareness, knowledge and understanding of body image so you can challenge the way you think and behave. Chapter 9 is dedicated to clinical disorders — what they are, recognising warning signs and where to go for help. There are some tips on how to tackle eating disorder behaviours such as binge eating. It is beyond the scope of this book to write about how to treat eating disorders, so suggestions are made as to where to go for help. This chapter also contains a section to assist parents and carers of children with their eating habits, including fussy eaters. For parents and teachers, you may like to go through the appendices work sheets together with your children.

People reading this book will be at different stages of readiness for change. You might simply be contemplating change, in which case take as much as you can in terms of an educational perspective so when you are ready you know what to do. Those who are ready for change and action, practice the activities as often as you can. It takes time to change and with all new skills it takes practice. At first it may be challenging but after a while it will get easier until you automatically know what to do when you catch yourself in a negative body image moment. For those who've already started their journey towards a positive body image, whether this is with a counsellor or health professional, use this book to enhance the work you're already doing.

Most people need to practice the techniques and strategies suggested in this book several times and for several weeks until they become automatic and a different way of thinking and behaving. So keep it up, even if you don't see changes right away. This book focuses on looking after yourself from head to toe, so use the tips to improve not just your body image but your whole self-image.

Most of all, enjoy your read and the activities. Stay positive, as believing that you can change the way you feel towards your body and the way you think about it will keep you motivated towards your goals. Loving the skin you're in is about body acceptance and celebrating diversity. Good luck and enjoy discovering a more positive way of seeing yourself and your body.

So let's get started!

Chapter 2

Goal setting

When I first went to see someone about my body image, my goal was to lose weight and be happy. I quickly learnt that my real goal was to feel contented in my life and with myself and that included my body image. And that in order to achieve this I actually had to stop focusing on losing weight. Losing weight never brought me happiness whereas learning to love and respect my body did.

Amanda, 27

When we want to change, we must have goals, things we can work towards and ways of measuring our success. In this section you'll learn how to set yourself some body image goals. This might seem basic but there's a bit of a knack to goal setting. How often have we set goals and never achieved them or given up half way there? Goals need to have a certain formula in order to ensure we keep motivated towards achieving them and see results from the start. This is called having SMART goals. By the end of this chapter, try and come up with your SMART goals and keep adding to them and crossing them off as you work through this book and begin to achieve them. Some goals will be ongoing such as 'feeling content with my body' and are achieved continuously; others will be more discrete.

When people are unhappy with their appearance they often try to change it through a wide range of behaviours. Such behaviours include dieting, excessive exercise, restricting food

intake and the use of a wide range of beauty regimes and products. Sometimes people even go to the more extreme measure
of seeking surgery in order to change their appearance. However,
research tells us that making changes to our physical appearance
including our weight will not always result in a more positive
body image. How many of us have set ourselves goals for weight
loss, only to either not achieve them and thus feel bad, or
achieved them and not feel any happier, or beating ourselves up
because we couldn't maintain them? Studies have shown, for
example, that losing weight or making other changes to our
appearance will not necessarily lead to improved body image or
feeling happier. So, when you're thinking about your goals, try
to make them about attitude change or engaging in healthier
behaviours rather than goals about changing your physical
appearance. Also, if we want to have long-term improvements in
our health and wellbeing, we need lifestyle change goals — these
are lifestyle goals we can maintain over the long term. For
example, regularly exercising or taking half an hour every day for
relaxation can be maintained long-term, whereas losing 10 kilos
or getting toned arms are very specific goals that can be achieved
in the short term but what can we work on in the long term?

Make your goals about attitude change

Try and think about goals that will achieve improvements in
how you feel about yourself and your body. These may not have
anything to do with changing how you actually look. If we focus
purely on changing the way we look, often these goals are unrealistic, unachievable and not maintainable. So, if goals around
changing our appearance will not necessarily result in a more
positive body image, then what will? Rather than taking steps
towards changing your physical appearance, the answer lies in
taking steps towards changing your *attitude* towards your appearance and yourself, the way you think about your body and self.
This change in thinking will have the effect of changing how you

feel towards your appearance and body and yourself. Remember here also, we're working on feeling better about ourselves inside and out, so think about lifestyle and health goals.

The way that your body looks on the outside does not have to influence the way that you feel about it on the inside. A great example is how some people who are born with disfiguring conditions can have a positive outlook on their life and those who might sustain disfigurements through burns or trauma can have little trouble adjusting to looking different (you may be interested in reading about the research being conducted at the Centre for Appearance Research in Bristol, UK). In contrast, there are people whose appearance we may idolise including celebrities who find it difficult to be happy with their looks despite having so called 'ideal' bodies. There are many examples of models and celebrities who talk about their battles with eating disorders and body image dissatisfaction and these are people whose bodies are supposed to be the 'ideal'. Your appearance does not mandate how you must feel about it. You can learn to accept your body, no matter what it looks like. Also, remember that no-one has a perfect body as there is no such thing. There may be people's bodies we admire or like the look of, but that doesn't mean we have to try and look like that and, let's face it, unless you've got the same genetic code it's virtually impossible anyway. You'll learn more about this in the following chapter that looks at societal body ideals.

It's also important when we're working on goals to focus on the positive. So, when we say to ourselves that we want to stop dieting or stop hating our body or stop obsessing about our receding hairline, it puts a negative spin on what we're trying to achieve. Rather than saying I want to stop such and such, it can be more helpful for us to focus on the positive. What do I want to do instead? For example, we might have a goal to look at ourselves in the mirror and focus on the things we like, to eat the things that are good for our body, to exercise for fun. So goals that tell us what we want to achieve and what we'll do instead of obsessive checking, for example, can help us focus on what we're trying to achieve rather than what we want to stop doing.

Our body image is personal and is based in experiences and influences which may be both unique or similar to others. While we might describe two people as both having a negative body image, their experiences are likely to be quite different. The parts of their body that they dislike will most likely differ along with the different events that trigger their distress. It is also likely that they have very different thoughts and feelings about their bodies and handle their problems in very different ways. It is often the importance we place on appearance, for example, that determines how our own perception will affect us. Therefore, your own body image experience is unique to you. The following chapter will help you see where your beliefs about and feelings towards your body may have come from, and in later chapters how you challenge these to feel more positive about your body.

It is worthwhile spending some time trying to understand your own body image, as the more we understand it, the easier it is to change. What parts of your body are you unhappy with? What situations trigger distress and lead you to feel negatively towards your body? What beliefs and assumptions do you have about your own body and about physical appearance in general and how do these affect the way you feel? What do you do to cope with these negative feelings? Answering such questions can not only assist you in understanding your current body image experience but can also help you identify particular areas that may be in need of change. It can be helpful when working on your goals to focus on how you'd like to feel, think and behave differently about and towards your body. For example, 'I'd like to feel more love towards my stomach, I'd like to stop overeating every day, and I'd like to exercise for fun'. Focus on what you'd like to do differently and put it in the positive. Remember to be specific and also think of how you'd measure the change, how you'd know when you've achieved your goals. There might some behaviours you'd like to increase such as fun activities and more exercise, and others you'd like to decrease such as overeating, starving yourself or exercising only for weight loss.

You might now like to think of 5–10 goals that you have around your body and how you feel about it, and keep referring back to them as you go through this book. A goal might be to stop worrying about your weight or stop feeling self-conscious when around others. Then write down how you'd know if you'd achieved this goal or not. For example, 'If I wasn't worried about my weight so much, I'd go out more with friends'. It's important to write down the ways you'd know if you'd achieved your goals so you can assess your progress as you move through the book.

Write these goals down and then as you go through the book write down how you would achieve these goals using the strategies and techniques.

When focusing on your goals, try and make them as specific as you can and write them in a way so that you would know whether you had achieved them or not. For example, you can see you have achieved the goal 'give my body one compliment per day' or 'feel less guilty about eating certain foods'. Also, make your goals achievable. It may be unrealistic to set yourself the goal to 'always feel positive about my body' or 'never eat bad foods'. Make sure your goals are achievable. And, so you can begin to see success straight away, you might want to set yourself some easier goals to start and then set goals that increase in difficulty. For example, you could set a goal first to better understand your own body image, learn techniques to overcome body image issues and then feel more positive about the part of your body you don't like.

So the key is to make your goals SMART, as I mentioned before. By SMART goals we mean the following:

S — Specific

Identify exactly what you want to see change in your attitude (how you feel, think and behave towards your body).

Remember, this book is not about changing your body — it's about changing how you feel, think and behave. For example, 'My goal is to appreciate what my body does for me in my daily life' is a bit general, but a specific goal would be to play netball with a group of girls for fun once a week. Another specific goal would be 'I want to feel comfortable when I'm wearing swimmers in the summer time when I'm at the beach'. To help you come up with specific goals, some questions to ask yourself are when, where, who, why?

M — Measurable

How will I know I've achieved my goal? What will I see, do, feel? For example, 'I will know I feel more positive towards my bottom by exercising for fun instead of to lose weight. I want to look at myself in the mirror and be able to list 10 positive things about it every day. The way I'll know I feel better in my body is because I will go to social events and not reject the invitation because I'm self-conscious of my body'. So, once you have your specific goal, write down how you will know you've achieved it. You might like to ask yourself how would someone else know you'd achieved your goal? What would they see?

A — Achievable

We all too often set goals that are too difficult to achieve; for example, 'I want to always feel good about my body'. This sort of goal is likely to be unrealistic as it's not really possible to feel good all the time. A more achievable goal might be 'to feel positive enough about my body that it doesn't stop me going swimming because I no longer feel self-conscious'. You can also set mini goals such as, 'This week I want to achieve this, in one month this and in a year this'. Think about what you can actually achieve and choose a time frame that is achievable. A few weeks is reasonable for behaviour change, or even right away. Thinking change will take much longer.

R — Realistic

As with achievable goals, don't set the bar too high. Make sure you write goals down that you know you can actually achieve, otherwise you'll only be disappointed and disheartened that you didn't achieve them. Set a mix of some easy and some more challenging goals. Maybe ask yourself, 'What can I achieve now, in a month, in a year, in three years?' By being realistic, I mean something that is within your reach. Try to make it about how you think, feel and behave rather than about changing your looks and appearance. For example, a lot of my clients want to stop worrying about their disliked body parts or want to feel good about their bodies. Many come to me with a goal to lose weight and I ask people to ask themselves, 'Why do I want to lose weight? What do I actually want?' If it's to feel fitter, feel more comfortable in your clothes, to be able to go to a party, to run around after the kids — then make these your goals. Remember, weight loss is only one way of measuring success in achieving health goals — there are lots of other ways such as through energy levels, cholesterol levels, lowered blood pressure, etc. So make this goal more specific rather than general.

T — Time

Set yourself a time frame for achievement of your goals and remember to be realistic. Don't set yourself a goal that you realistically can't achieve in a short period of time. For example, if you want to lower your cholesterol levels or blood pressure, you will need to set other goals which will lead to the achievement of your health goal and it may take some months until you've achieved it.

ACTIVITY

Ask yourself the question: 'What are my SMART body image goals?' Turn to Appendix A for a help sheet on setting goals.

CHAPTER SUMMARY

▌ Focus on changing your attitude towards your appearance rather than changing your actual appearance.

▌ Changing your attitude will lead to positive body image.

▌ Focus on the changes you need to make to your behaviour and way of thinking in order to feel more positive about your body and self.

▌ Write down your goals in the positive: What do I want to be doing? How do I want to be thinking?

▌ Make your goals SMART goals.

Now that you have identified your goals, let's start looking at body image and where our perceptions of our bodies and selves comes from. At any stage in this book you can revisit your goals, revise as needed and also tick off as you achieve them. Chapter 14 talks about the importance of rewards for goal achievement so you may like to have a look at this chapter too.

Chapter 3

What is body image and what is its significance?

I grew up thinking my body was ugly. I was teased at school because I was shorter and plumper than the other children. I used to cry and tell my mum. She put me on a diet to try and lose weight, thinking this would solve the problem. I felt ashamed of my body because my friends didn't like it and now neither did my mum. The dieting just made me eat more, but in secret. So I got fatter and felt worse about my body and myself. The teasing continued until I left school. I hated school. As an adult I overate, especially when I felt bad. I went to see a psychologist who helped me identify why I felt the way I did towards my body and how to change my relationship with my body and learn who I am as a person. I learnt that my adult perception was based on how I thought others perceived me. I have my own perception now, based on the real me, my talents, qualities and who I am as a person. Now when I feel bad I don't turn to food; I turn to my true friends who love me for me.

Jody, 25

What do we mean by the term 'body image'?

Body image is a broad term that relates to a person's perceptions of and 'attitudes and feelings towards' their physical appearance. For example, do you like the parts of your body? Do you feel positively towards the parts of your body? Do you feel good in your skin? The way that you perceive your body may not always be the same as others perceive it. For example, when looking in the mirror you may perceive the size of your hips to be larger than they actually are, or larger than other people actually perceive them. This is because our perception is distorted by many things such as the influences in our life, our mood, the other things we're thinking about, how rested or tired we are, and what we've eaten, among many, many other factors. So, often what we see in the mirror isn't our true reflection — it's our perception of our reflection, and this can change. It's quite common, for example, for partners to comment on how beautiful or attractive their partner is but for this partner not to believe it. This is because our partners and friends see us for our qualities and positive elements, whereas we are often much harsher judges of ourselves, especially if we're feeling depressed or down. We also look at ourselves with all of our prior experiences, both positive and negative, and these influence our picture of ourselves. We often are our worst enemies and the harshest judges of our bodies. If only we could see the beauty that others see.

Beauty is in the eye of the beholder. And you hold the key to your own body love and confidence.

Body image also incorporates thoughts, or the things you tell yourself about your body, along with the assumptions you may hold about physical appearance and what you should look like or what you consider is true beauty. The thoughts and assumptions you have about your body and physical appearance generate feelings about your body. For example, you may have the thought, 'I really like the way I look in these pants today', which will lead to positive feelings towards your body. Alternatively, you may have the thought, 'My arms are so flabby, I am sure everyone in the room is staring at them. I really should spend more time at the gym', which will lead to negative feelings towards your body. Why are some people affected by their body image to the point where how they feel about their body affects their day-to-day life and others don't seem to care? A lot lies in the importance we place on appearance, weight and shape. For example, if my self-esteem is built on my family and career and they're going well, then I'll feel good; if on the other hand my self-esteem is built on being thin and I perceive that I'm fat, then I won't feel very good at all. And this feeling bad will likely lead me to stop doing things that make me feel good.

Body Dysmorphic Disorder

Let's talk briefly here about an extreme body image disorder that has a clinical diagnosis. Body Dysmorphic Disorder (BDD) is a disorder where a person is preoccupied with an imagined or exaggerated perception of a particular defect in their appearance. Often there is nothing wrong at all with the person's appearance but they perceive that there is. Typically a person may be excessively concerned about the shape of a facial feature, hairline, or other part of their body such as genitals. This preoccupation causes the person much distress and they typically spend a large amount (usually hours) of time checking and re-checking this body part. It causes the person impairment socially and occupationally, usually because they are self-conscious and distracted by constant thoughts about the body part. It is not to be mistaken with a preoccupation with weight or shape as seen in the eating disorders.

If you feel you are suffering from BDD you are best advised to seek professional assistance. There is a list of places to get help at the end of this book. Seeing your general practitioner for a referral is a good first point of call. This disorder can be treated and the sufferer should not be ashamed to discuss this with a health professional as it is a very real condition that needs to be taken seriously because it causes significant impairment to a person's life.

The effects of having a negative body image

Having a negative body image can lead to many negative consequences such as engagement in behaviours that are harmful to
our health as well as feelings of anxiety and depression. This is
because the way we're thinking leads us to behave in ways consistent with this. For example, if we're thinking we're not good
at something, we're less likely to do it. We also tend to do things
that reinforce this negative thinking. When we're thinking a
negative thought such as we're fat and fat is ugly, we're likely to
stay at home, isolate ourselves and do things that make us feel
fatter and uglier. Therefore, tackling the problem can lead to
feeling and thinking differently as this improves our self-esteem,
mood, sexual fulfilment and general wellbeing. The effects of
having a negative body image, on the other hand, can affect the
way we see yourselves overall. Feeling unhappy with part of your
body or its size and shape can lead to feelings of unhappiness
generally, thinking no-one will like me if I look this way. For
some people who are concerned about their weight, the number
on the scales in the morning can have such a significant effect
that it determines whether they will have a good or bad day.

How we feel about our body can also cause us a lot of
anxiety. For example, when we might be self-conscious and so
keep checking our hair or clothing and worry about how we
look. It's common for people with body image concerns to
worry a lot of the day about their appearance, such as their
weight, what they've eaten, how much exercise they've done,
and this leads to a lot of unhappiness. I've seen men with concerns about hair loss, for example, spend hours checking their
scalp and hair for evidence of loss, to the point where they may
not be able to leave the house. Worrying about what others may
see causes them enormous anxiety which disrupts their concentration and enjoyment of social activities.

It's quite common for adolescents to spend quite a bit of
time getting ready and on their appearance including checking

their hair, skin and body. So, if you're a parent or carer reading this book for your adolescent, remember that this is normal behaviour. What indicates concern is if they are spending hours on their appearance and not feeling good about it. They're becoming distressed by their appearance or it's impacting on the other things in their lives. Adolescence is a time of change and where appearance issues can be very important and quite distressing if not 'just right'. Remember that our appearance is just one part of who we are and it doesn't define us unless we let it. Sometimes as adolescents we can get caught up in our appearance being the be all and end all, and become upset if it's not right and how we want it to be. If you're an adolescent reading this book, remember that there are many things that make you important in your life and the lives of those around you. It can help to think, 'What is it my friends and family like about me?' You can bet it's not appearance related. Use this book to help you reduce the importance you place on your appearance so you can open your eyes to the wonderful world of you.

ACTIVITY

Write down what are the qualities that make you unique? What do friends and family like about you? If you don't know, ask!

Feelings of masculinity and femininity can be influenced by our body image too. Some people believe that, if they don't have the physical qualities such as muscles for men or thinness for women that they associate with being masculine or feminine, then they feel less of a person and that they're not truly identified as a man or woman. These negative feelings of masculinity or femininity can affect a person's interactions with potential sexual mates as well as sexual performance and enjoyment.

How we feel about our bodies also effects our interactions with others. How many of us haven't gone out with friends because we don't think we look good enough or aren't confident enough about how we look? Being self-conscious about our physical appearance can also affect how intimate we are in our relationships. For example, feeling so self-conscious that we can't enjoy the experience or even avoiding being naked or putting our body on show even with the person we love.

Where body concerns are significant is where we see eating disorders such as Anorexia Nervosa and Bulimia Nervosa. These are clinical conditions that significantly affect a person's wellbeing both physically and psychologically. There is a special section in this book dedicated to understanding eating disorders and where to go for help.

A negative body image (i.e., not being happy with the way you look) can lead people to feel depressed, anxious and self-conscious around others, and limit themselves socially, in relationships, at school or work and in their family life. Those with a positive body image, on the other hand, can feel self-confident and this may enhance their feelings about themselves and their lives and lead them to engage in more activities with others. This difference often depends on the importance people attribute to their looks. For example, someone who does not see their looks as being important would not be affected by whether they like how they look or not. This is significant in terms of prevention and intervention in that we need to promote other qualities other than looks and attractiveness being tied to success in Westernised societies.

Body image is a serious clinical issue, as a negative body image (for example, perceiving oneself as fat, when you are not) is one of the criteria for the eating disorder anorexia. It has been shown to influence both adult men and women's behaviour as well as children's, including dieting and exercise behaviour as well as more dangerous practices such as diet pills, steroid use and purging. People may even go to the extreme of undergoing plastic surgery to remove or change a 'perceived' defect in their appearance. We also know that children as young as seven can have body image disturbances leading them to developing eating disorders. There comes an emphasis on body image particularly as girls begin puberty. Some girls will embrace this and be proud of their more womanly shape, whereas others will shy away, doing all that they can to try and 'stop' this natural process (e.g., through extreme dieting, covering up their curves and developing breasts, and avoiding swimming).

How many people are affected by body image concerns and why?

> *I wish my body looked like the models I see on the shows I watch. I want to be tall and skinny cos that's beautiful and everyone likes you if you look like that. I have been on a few diets and I am currently cutting out carbs to not get fat. My friends at school are also dieting. I don't like going swimming because I worry about my bum and legs looking too fat.*
>
> *Sarina, 10.*

Concerns with the body are occurring in younger and younger age groups. We know that children as young as seven have developed eating disorders. Girls like Sarina can develop body image concerns because of the comparisons they make with others their age, learning from parents, learning from exposure to media messages promoting thinness, and media associations with dieting and perceived happiness and success.

About one-third of men are unhappy with their bodies and about two-thirds of women experience body dissatisfaction, whether that is with the body as a whole or particular parts. We know that primary-school-aged children can experience body dissatisfaction and even start to diet at this young age. Eating disorders are rare in children but children do engage in body change behaviours such as dieting and exercising for appearance reasons, including muscle building in boys. Eating disorders in women occur in about 2–3% of the Western population and about one in 10 of these are men.

Although the incidence of eating disorders marked by extreme forms of body dissatisfaction have remained fairly stable, body image concerns are on the rise, particularly for men and boys. It's still the case that a negative body image affects more women than men; this is likely due to more emphasis placed on appearance in women and the body 'ideal' being that of thinness, a thinness 99% of women cannot achieve without significantly affecting their health and wellbeing. The internalisation or acceptance of this 'thin ideal' is a risk factor for body image disturbance including development of Anorexia Nervosa. As well, this 'thin ideal' is far more entrenched in women, with a greater intensity to live up to this ideal than the 'muscular ideal' for men. However, body image dissatisfaction has increased for men. This is possibly due to the change in the representation of the ideal male now being one of the 'metrosexual' (fit, slim, toned physique) which, as for women, very few men without significant dieting and the hiring of a personal trainer plus use of expensive and often dangerous products could achieve.

As we will talk about in the next chapter, understanding what influences the way we feel and the thoughts we have about our bodies and the assumptions and beliefs we have about physical appearance can help us challenge them and change to feel more positive about our bodies and selves. By taking steps towards changing these things, we can go a long way towards enhancing our body image.

Research on male body image in Australia

Recently, there has been an increasing recognition that men and boys experience dissatisfaction with their physiques and that body dissatisfaction is not just a female issue. It is believed that Western men's body image dissatisfaction has tripled in the last 25 years, from 15% to 45% in Australia, for example. As is the case for women, men's body dissatisfaction has been linked to a number of potentially serious health consequences including anxiety over eating and eating disorders, excessive exercise, steroid use, depression and low self-esteem. Alarmingly, it is estimated that one in four Australian men in the healthy weight range believe themselves to be fat, while 17% of men are on a weight-loss diet, 20% of regular exercisers are addicted to exercise and around 3% use muscle-enhancing drugs. Moreover, a recent survey by Mission Australia revealed that for young adult males body image was the second greatest concern behind alcohol use. While it is clear that men are experiencing body dissatisfaction, the scientific research on the body image concerns of men is limited and inconsistent.

We often stigmatise body image as being a women's issue or indicative of 'girlishness' in men. It is important to recognise that men and boys just like girls and women worry about their appearance and bodies. For example, a recent survey on males aged 12–25 conducted by Mission Australia showed that body image concerns were at the top, above family, friends, relationship and school and work concerns. Men often worry about their weight and their muscularity, particularly the upper body. Men often deny worrying about their appearance — it isn't seen as appropriate for men to discuss body image with each other, often with fear of being labelled as 'girlie'. So who do men go to if not their mates for help?

Many men want to change their bodies. They believe that if they change how they look they'll feel better, be more popular with the ladies, get a promotion etc. However, changing your body through modifying weight, purchasing protein shakes, getting hair plugs etc. makes men temporarily feel better but it doesn't actually improve their quality of life or long-term happiness.

Men very rarely seek help for body image concerns, especially from a professional, but are generally willing to talk to a fitness instructor or trainer. Men rarely talk to each other about their appearance concerns, often seeing it as 'sissy'. This therefore means that a lot of men are worrying about their bodies without having an outlet to express this and without getting the help they need.

This book will hopefully help those men who might be worrying in secret about their bodies.

It's interesting to note that, when asked, women often prefer a man who is a lot less muscular then men think women desire. Many studies in Australia and overseas have found this to be the case, that it is men, more so than women who desire muscularity in men. This desire for muscularity exists all over the world. Along with this desire is a misperception of actual appearance, with men often perceiving themselves to be less muscular and slightly fatter than they actually are, making their dissatisfaction with their appearance more significant. So, like women, men are also not very accurate when judging their own physiques.

Men often idealise these muscular physiques because of their association with desirable traits such as masculinity and success. Previously this could have been achieved through the workplace or their role as breadwinner in the family. Now, in modern society, women have unprecedented access into previously male dominated areas such as business, academia and the defence forces and have increased their earning potential. This change is closing the gap between men and women in terms of career and finances with the effect of some men turning to appearance change as a marker of masculinity.

The muscular, lean, toned physique for men is also associated with being advantageous in courting potential partners and in sexual performance, making this physique more desirable. The same occurs for women, where the thin ideal is associated with success, male attention, attractiveness and wealth. When we associate a certain body with desirable traits it's not surprising we'll desire to have this body type and work on trying to achieve it. What's important to realise is that it's ok to admire certain physiques, just like we might admire certain qualities and talents, but that doesn't mean we should compare ourselves in a negative way. Just because we don't have the physique or qualities we admire doesn't make us less of a person or ugly or deficit in comparison. We are unique and there are many things about us that others may admire without us even knowing but we wouldn't expect others to try and look and be like us would we?

It's ok to admire other's bodies, but it's the taking on board of this thinking that we're less in comparison, and working to try and achieve a different body in a way that's detrimental to our health and wellbeing, that needs our attention. Remember, the images we see in the media are just that, images — they're not real people, and having that physique may be associated with desirable qualities but it certainly doesn't guarantee it and there are many ways to achieve success, health, happiness, attraction and improved sexual perform-ance without doing anything appearance-related.

What are the benefits of a positive body image?

I'm beautiful because I have a nice smile and I'm kind and nice to my friends and my pet dog. I like jumping on my trampoline and going to sleep overs with friends from school. I'm good at English and the piano. I like school and doing craft. I like it when my mum brushes my hair and I like wearing my favourite colour. My body is special to me as it helps me do the things I like and keeps me healthy. I really like my arms at the moment because they're strong enough to help me hold my new baby sister.

Sarah, 8

Having a positive perception of our bodies enhances our self-esteem — our feelings about ourselves overall. We're more likely to behave in ways that are good for our health and wellbeing when we feel positive about our bodies. We're also more likely to engage with the world around us when we feel positive and confident in our skin. Being healthy and taking care of ourselves and our wellbeing is more likely to occur when we value our bodies. We feel more comfortable socially and in public and are more likely to jump in there and do things when we feel good about our bodies.

Now we understand what body image is and the sorts of ideals that men and women have, as well as some of the consequences to mind and body of a negative body image, we can now look at why it is that we idealise these figures and start to look at how we change our perceptions and the way we view our bodies in order to have a more positive image of ourselves. The first step in changing our body image is understanding where our beliefs have come from.

CHAPTER SUMMARY

▪ Body image is a perception, attitude and feeling towards our physical appearance as a whole and its parts.

▪ Our body image is influenced by our past experiences, mood, importance placed on appearance, and self-esteem.

▪ Body Dysmorphic Disorder and eating disorders are clinical disorders associated with body image disturbance and are treatable.

▪ Our body image affects our behaviour and how we feel about ourselves.

▪ Body image disturbance affects men and women of all ages.

▪ Men need to come forward with their body image issues and not be afraid to ask for help.

▪ We can achieve success, happiness, wealth, sexual attraction, and many, many other qualities without changing our appearance at all.

▪ A positive body image can improve our self-esteem, mood, confidence and enjoyment in life.

Parts of this chapter have been published in *InPsych*, the Bulletin of the Australian Psychological Society Limited, August 2012©The Australian Psychological Society Limited and is available online at www.psychology.org.au/inpsych/.

Chapter 4

The development of a negative body image and overcoming it

I love my body and I thank my mum for this. She always told me I was beautiful just like her and my sister. My mum used to say it was my caring nature that shone on the outside, that my smile was like turning on a light, bright and comforting. When I went through puberty I experienced some teasing from my peers because I was bigger than the other girls. This made me feel bad about my body at times. But my mum would tell me that the bullies were focusing on my size which was just one part of me and not me as a whole. She was a big believer in celebrating body diversity. My mum helped me get through what was a tough time at school. She was always a good role model.

Sandra, 17

In the previous chapter we talked about what is body image — that it's a perception of our physical selves, what we think we look like, our like or dislike of it as a whole or its parts. Body image is also about thoughts — what we think about our body and subsequently how we feel towards it. It is these feelings about our body and our selves that cause people the most unhappiness, anxiety and distress and it is these feelings that lead us to engage in behaviours which may help or hinder. In this chapter you will learn about the development of body image, as it is understanding where our body image beliefs and thoughts come from that will help us understand the way we think and learn to think differently in order to feel better about our body and ourselves. Here you'll be introduced to the ABCs of body image and then in the next chapter we'll start working on how we change our behaviour and thoughts to feel better about our bodies and ourselves.

The ABCs of body image

If I asked you to tell me how you think about your body you'd probably tell me something about how you feel towards it. So let me start by distinguishing thoughts from feelings. When we're in a situation, at a social event for example, we can usually recount the way we feel. Perhaps we feel anxious or uncomfortable or perhaps we feel happy and excited. We may therefore say it was because of the social event that we feel the way we do. However, what actually makes us feel the way we feel is our thoughts. This explains why two people can be in the same situation but have completely different experiences. The event is the same but their feelings are different and this is because of their thoughts. Let me use an example. Two girls are at the beach, both sunbaking and sitting on the sand. Girl one feels incredibly self-conscious in her swimmers but girl two doesn't. The event is the same but they feel differently. Why? Because their thoughts are different. Girl one is thinking, 'I look fat in my swimsuit, I have a horrible body', whereas girl two is thinking, 'I am happy with my body the way it is, what a lovely sunny day'.

Using the ABC model, we call the A the *antecedent* (or event), the B is our *beliefs* (or thoughts) and the C is the *consequence* (feelings and behaviour). We all too often think A leads to C but in fact it's the B, our beliefs and thoughts, that lead to feelings. In Chapter 5 and 6 we will learn about how to change our thoughts and beliefs in order to feel better as well as changing our behaviour. But for now let's focus on the influence of A, the antecedent and its effect on our thinking.

A

Antecedents (events) and the development of a negative body image

There are many theories about how a negative body image develops. By negative we mean a dislike for your body as a whole or parts of it, and perceiving it to be ugly or needing change. The development of body image whether positive or negative takes time to develop and it starts developing from a very young age even before we start school — think of the influence of parents and the programs children watch. Our experiences throughout life help shape the formation of our beliefs and thoughts about our bodies and ourselves. It is often a combination of factors that determines our body image. No one factor alone influences our body image. I often have parents ask if they caused their child's eating disorder for example, and the answer is not a simple 'yes'. There are many, many things that lead a person to develop an eating disorder. Let's go through a few influences now. Understanding where your body image perception comes from, how it developed and what's maintaining it will help you understand your current body image. And when we can understand our own body image, how it developed and what's perhaps maintaining our beliefs and the way we feel, we're much better able to change it.

Knowledge and insight helps us understand ourselves and make positive change if we need it.

How much our body image affects our daily life depends on many factors, including how important our body image is to us. Now's a good time to evaluate how much importance you place on your body image. Think of all the things in your life

---

ACTIVITY

Think about how much importance do I place on my body image. Why do I place this much importance on it? Is this helpful? or do I need to try and reduce the importance I place on my appearance in order to feel better? — You will learn how to do this in the next few chapters.

Understanding your body image and its development will help you to make positive changes.

---

and what you're doing and place body image within them. It'll be good to reflect later in this book as to whether you change how important it is in your life. The importance a person places on appearance and the context in which the body is seen often determine how much their body image affects their life.

An important part of changing our body image is first understanding how it has come to develop in the first place and what factors affect it. If we can understand the origins of where our beliefs about and attitudes towards our bodies come from, it can help to explain why we've arrived at this place now of disliking our bodies. As we talked about in the previous chapter, it is our beliefs about our bodies that influence our behaviour and feelings. So, if we challenge our beliefs, we can change the way we feel and behave. Sound simple? Well, it's not. Be prepared for a challenge. If it was simple, you would have done it a long time ago. Beliefs take time to develop and therefore changing them will take time as well. We basically have to learn to think about our bodies and selves differently.

A — The influence of the culture we live in

The way male and female bodies are portrayed in the media, whether that be magazines, television or the internet, shape our perceptions about what our bodies 'should' look like and we receive these messages from a very early age. There are certain cultural body ideals that exist in all cultures. The way the human body is portrayed gives us a point of comparison for our own body. It is this comparison that often leads us to feel positive or negative towards our body. For example, if we compare ourselves to an ideal image portrayed in the media, then we're much more likely to think of our body in negative terms in comparison. Unfortunately this negative perception is very common when we compare ourselves to what are unrealistic images in the media. For example, in Western society today there is a tendency to highly value thinness in women, seeing a thin woman as associated often with success, attention and wealth. And for men this ideal image is a lean and muscular figure, characterised as leading to the attraction of women, wealth, success and pride. Both 'ideals' (what society says is most attractive) are almost impossible for most people to achieve, yet we are bombarded every day with images of film stars and fashion models that are often dangerously thin and we are fed a message that thin is beautiful or that a real man should be lean and full of muscles. These media images also centre on youthfulness so as we age we move further and further away from these ideals which can lead us to feel unhappy as we age naturally. Being realistic about making comparisons to these images is important. There's no point trying to look much younger than we actually are. We might be able to look youthful, but if we're in our 40s, for example, comparing ourselves to a late-teen image is only going to make us feel dissatisfied with our appearance in comparison.

As was discussed in the previous chapter, these unrealistic images of thinness for women and leanness and muscularity for men have seen dramatic increases in negative body image and eating disorders in Western society. This negative body image can occur for people at all ages — there are cases of women in their

50s and 60s with eating disorders. This is because we strive for these idealised images because of the positivity and normalisation we see attached to them. This is in contrast to societies where food is scarce: a full figured female and heavier body for both men and women is the ideal and this is related to lower incidence of dieting, exercising for fat loss and eating disorders. What happens when we see these media images is that we internalise them ('I must look like that'), and therefore strive to attain something that is unattainable. Because it is unattainable it often leads us, particularly women, to engage in dangerous dieting and eating behaviours, working hard to never actually achieve the goal. Not attaining this goal then leads to a negative perception of oneself, negative beliefs and thoughts and therefore feelings of sadness and dislike for the body and self. This striving for idealised images can also explain the use of beauty products such as supposed anti-ageing creams, hair colouring and hair loss treatment.

Why, though, do we take so much notice of the media and let it influence our thoughts about ourselves? We're bombarded by idealised images everywhere we go, so it's very hard to avoid them. It's often this overwhelming push of certain figures, seeing them over and over again, that leads us to naturally compare ourselves, see a difference, and see a fault in our own body in comparison.

So how do we stop being influenced by these media images? In essence we need to realise that real bodies don't look anything like what is portrayed in the media. For example, in magazines, the images we see are not the true person at all but rather an air-brushed, computer enhanced, touched-up version of the person with no imperfections. Understanding media images, often called media literacy, will help you to stop comparing yourself to unrealistic images in the media. Knowing that these images are unrealistic and unachievable will help you to stop aspiring to look like them. The supermodel Cindy Crawford once said, 'Even I don't wake up in the morning looking like

Cindy Crawford'. Here she was making a point about how all of her pictures in magazines are digitally enhanced even after full make-up, air-brushing and other cosmetic procedures.

Celebrating our age, our maturity, our growth of knowledge and wisdom as we get older is another way to not fall victim to trying to move our bodies in line with idealised images. Being happy with oneself is about celebrating the years we have and appreciating ourselves at any age and stage of life.

> *I just turned 70 and celebrated my life to date with friends and family. I'm blessed with all the experiences I've had and all the people in my life. Sure, my skin is wrinkly, I'm carrying more weight than I did when I was in my twenties and I have grey hair, but that's what real women my age look like as far as I'm concerned. My husband tells me how much he loves my body because when he looks at me it reminds him of the children we've had together and the happy times we've had. He wouldn't swap me for a younger version because that version wouldn't be the same person I am now.*
>
> *Joanne*

Chapter 13 on children's body image and being a good role model will talk about media literacy in detail. As an adult we may decide we need to stop buying certain magazines or watching certain shows if we find they lead us to become more negative about our bodies or more distressed as we compare ourselves to people in them. You might like to identify things you read or watch that actually cause you distress or anxiety, making your body image worse. You may need to stop engaging in these

---

ACTIVITY

Ask yourself: 'What are the things I read or watch that lead me to feel negative about my body?' Do I need to change or stop bombarding myself with those negative influences?

behaviours as part of improving your attitude and positive feelings towards your body.

As we've just stated, societal 'ideals' (what the media says is attractive) also exist for men. Often a lot of attention is paid to women, but for men their images are unrealistic also. Not only is the supposed ideal male image very fit, with no body fat and very successful, but he has little body hair, a full head of hair and is young. This is completely unrealistic for boys to achieve before puberty as well as for older men. While for women the ideal body shape is thin, for men it is muscular. Muscular chests and arms, strong facial features and a full head of hair are the cultural ideal. Often men jeopardise their health through behaviours such as the use of steroids or excessive exercise in order to reach this ideal. As well, men can engage in starving themselves and alternatively binge eating just like women. There's also a trend for men to spend a lot of money on beauty treatments such as waxing and other products in order to look a certain way. There's nothing wrong with doing things that make your body feel nice, but always ask yourself, 'Does this make me feel good or does it feed my anxiety and make me more self-conscious?'

> I used to think that I exercised to be healthy and to feel good.
> But I really did it to try and stop feeling anxious. But then I
> realised that exercising was feeding my anxiety as I was doing it
> only to stop gaining weight. If I missed a day or didn't work
> out as hard as I'd planned, I'd feel depressed and even more
> anxious about working harder the next day. I developed a
> problem with over-exercising where I felt anxious all of the time.
>
> Tom, 32

Western society ideals of beauty are unrealistic and for most of us unachievable. While we may not have the power to change society's ideals, we do have the power to decide whether we buy into them or not. Society's standards can't harm you unless you buy into them and by holding more realistic ideals ourselves we can improve our body image.

An activity to help understand outside influences on body image is to think about what the outside perceptions or pressures of female/male ideals might be and then think how it makes you feel about yourself given this pressure. Then think about how you would like females/males to be seen in society — what would be valued by society and then how you would feel about yourself if society valued you in this different way. Societal change only comes from us challenging perceptions and values. This is a great activity for teachers to do with children and adolescents to teach them about questioning media images.

As we will discuss in the coming chapter, the only way to not fall victim to media and societal pressure is to challenge these media images and the value placed on looks. Perhaps you could start looking at people differently too. Look out for the qualities and non-appearance-related attributes that you like in someone. The more you practice doing this with others, the easier it will be to do this with yourself.

A — The influence of other significant people in our lives— parents, peers and other family members

Throughout our lives family and friends can also have a significant impact on our body image. For example, we may have grown up in a family that places a great amount of emphasis on physical appearance and losing weight or looking a particular way. We may also be influenced through watching the behaviour of our family members. For example, watching a parent or sibling constantly complain about their looks can have an impact on how much emphasis we place on the importance of physical appearance. Seeing our beautiful mother call herself ugly or fat can make us grow up thinking there's something wrong with the way we look. After all, aren't we a genetic makeup of her?

Other things we can learn from our mothers are our relationships with food. Seeing our mothers dieting and not eating certain foods can set up food rules for us about good and bad foods, often leading us to feel guilty if we eat them. Sometimes it can be our upbringing that influences our relationship with food — where we've been taught certain food rules as children, we can often carry these through into adulthood. It can be good to reflect here about the foods you do and don't eat and why. Then ask yourself whether this is relevant and healthy for you now. Sometimes fussy adult eaters can have developed food aversions as children and carry this through to adulthood. As you'll learn in Chapter 8, when there are behaviours we engage in that are unhelpful or prohibit us from enjoying life, we may have to challenge our food rules and experiment with breaking them.

Sometimes men can become overly concerned with the way they look as adults because they've been teased about being overweight as children or because relatives have made comments about them putting on weight. Comments from peers about being scrawny or weedy can lead males to feel very unhappy with their appearance and also lead some to feel less masculine or effective as a man. Here's an example of how Bob felt:

> *I felt like less of a man because I didn't have big muscles as an adolescent and young man and carried this through into middle age. Now I think what a waste, all that stress over my looks and it didn't get me ahead. In fact it held me back because I was so self-conscious at times that I didn't do the things that may have got me ahead in life.*
>
> *Bob, 45*

There is also a significant amount of evidence that suggests being teased about our appearance, whether it be by family members or friends, can greatly impact on our body image. People who report being teased about their physical appearance as children and adolescents are more likely to be dissatisfied with the way they look as adults. It's a horrible thing being teased and it's hard not to take it personally and internalise it as being our true self. Remember that it's common for people to be teased and the easiest thing to tease people about is their appearance because it's more obvious than their talents and traits. This doesn't make it true. Our appearance changes rapidly as we age and particularly as we go through puberty. So what we were teased for as an adolescent is likely to no longer be relevant as an adult.

This will be discussed more later in the book, but the main way to overcome our adult negative body image is to work out what started this perception and then ask ourselves is this valid or relevant to us now? It's called disputing our thoughts through looking for evidence against our way of thinking.

A — Another influence: Our personality

There are some personality characteristics such as having low self-esteem or being a perfectionist — where everything has to be just right or completely 'correct' — that can affect body image. A great sense of achievement can come out of achieving a weight-loss goal or toning-up an area of the body, but sometimes this can turn into an obsession where the change is never good enough. This can lead people to feel very unhappy accompanied with feelings of failure for never achieving the 'perfect' body. One thing we can do is look at our own standards for beauty and try and reassess them to be more realistic. Ask yourself, 'If I don't expect others to live up to these standards, then why do I expect myself to live up to these standards? Is it my perfectionism that's getting in the way of my happiness with my body? How can I accept myself as I am and even love my perceived imperfections?' Many of my clients with anorexia set themselves very high standards of they must be thin, and if not, they are no good. I get them to ask themselves what makes a worthwhile person? When they start to answer, they invariably start to list qualities and traits which they themselves have. I ask them to revaluate themselves without thinness as the ideal goal. Here's an example from Chloe:

I thought thin women had it all. I saw thin models in magazines and thought, 'I want that. I want to be successful, happy, popular and sexy'. I spent two years trying to achieve this. I certainly achieved thinness but I didn't experience the success and happiness I expected. Instead I developed an eating disorder and depression. I had to stop school and I lost a lot of friends. I went into therapy and learnt to see myself for my talents, personality, traits, hobbies and abilities. I gained my weight back but I didn't care because I'd also regained myself and the best parts of me!

Chloe, 17

A — What's influencing you right now?

While past experiences at school and home and influences of people and events can impact on body image, even more important are the influences currently affecting us, those that are maintaining the way we feel about our bodies. Who and what is influencing you now? For adults, ask yourself why you continue to have the same perception you may have had when you were younger. For adolescents, ask yourself what is influencing your body image right now. Is it your friends? What you watch or read?

It is important to gain an understanding of the influences from our past; however, blaming them for body image problems won't help solve them. In order to make any kind of change to our body image, we need to understand the things currently influencing it. For example, are we holding onto teasing about our weight as a child and worried about returning to that? Are we trying to make our body look a certain way because a previous partner made a comment? Are we desperately trying to get our body to look like it did in our youth?

Understanding the situations that trigger our body image distress and anxiety is important, along with understanding the thoughts and beliefs that these situations may trigger. It is also important to understand the consequences of these thoughts and beliefs (i.e., the feelings we have and the behaviours we engage in) when trying to understand those influences currently impacting on body image. Let's look now at what's currently happening for us that is triggering our body image beliefs.

Often in our daily lives we may encounter situations that lead to the activation of our negative body image thoughts and beliefs which we've developed as a consequence of our past. These situations vary from person to person but can include such situations as seeing someone who we think is attractive, catching a glimpse of our reflection in the mirror, hopping on the scales or trying on new clothes. Such situations can be very distressing for people with a negative body image and can trigger a wide range of negative body image thoughts and beliefs. This is where we may decide to stop these triggers if we can, or replace them with more helpful behaviours or ways of thinking.

For adolescents, your peer group may be a big source of body anxiety. This is a time of life where appearance focus is quite intense as you're going through so many changes to your body, brain, learning and hormones, as well as trying to work out who you are, your identity. So it's understandable you may try to define yourself through your looks. But remember this is just one part of you and a part of you that is constantly changing through life. Focusing on what makes you aside from your appearance is a good way to feel good about yourself. Ask yourself what do my friends like about me? What talents do I have? What things do I enjoy? If there are situations or people that make you feel negative about your body and self, then you may need to limit your contact with these people or learn strategies for handling these situations such as being assertive. The next three chapters will help with strategies for dealing with difficult people.

Chapter 7 will look at how you can challenge your thinking and beliefs, but let's just touch on it briefly here.

> Write down here some of your triggers for negative body image. What situations lately have you caught yourself in where your negative body image has been activated? Why is this? What thoughts do these situations trigger? Then turn to the next chapters to work on challenging your thinking to feel better.

B

Beliefs and thoughts

Now let's turn to looking at our beliefs (thoughts) and how these influence our body image. As I mentioned before, it's not the event that triggers the feeling but our thoughts about the event. Often these thoughts happen so quickly that we don't notice this important step and so just assume that an event has led to a feeling. We often call these *automatic thoughts*, as they can occur in milliseconds and we're often not consciously aware of them. If we can slow this process down, though, and become more conscious of it, we're much better able to control and change it. Being aware of our negative self-talk allows us to work on changing it to be more balanced and positive.

Thoughts triggered regarding our body can vary from negative self-talk such as 'People are going to look at me and not like what they see' to generalised appearance beliefs and assumptions such as 'I'm too fat to be liked' or 'I can't go to the gym until I lose weight' or 'I'm too bald for a woman to find me attractive'. Such thoughts can have huge consequences on the way we feel and the things we do. Have a think about some of the things you say to yourself in regards to your appearance. You may need to spend some time becoming aware of your thoughts and self-talk. Be on the lookout for your thoughts and write them down when you catch them. By becoming more aware of them, you're much more able to challenge and change them! We will look at challenging or disputing our thoughts and appearance assumptions in Chapter 7 in more detail. This is just a taste.

ACTIVITY

Ask yourself: 'What thoughts and beliefs do you have that lead you to feel negative about your body? Are they specific thoughts or generalised beliefs?'

I always thought I felt a particular way, such as lonely, and so that's why I overate. Then I realised it was actually my thoughts that were making me overeat. I'd feel lonely or down and so I'd start telling myself I was hopeless and my life was going nowhere so I might as well overeat and feel disgusting to match how I thought about myself. Things started to turn around when I learnt to value and respect myself. When I thought to myself, 'You're important and overeating will just make you feel worse, and I could do something else instead', I started to feel better and overeating slowly began to lose its place in my life.

Donna, 44.
Suffered from depression and binge eating disorder

C
Consequences — Feelings and behaviours

We feel what we think, and subsequently one of the consequences of thinking negatively about our bodies is to feel negatively about it. For example, if you tell yourself, 'Everyone will thinking I'm ugly until I lose weight', then you'll likely feel bad about your appearance and low in mood. Or, if you tell yourself, 'No girl will want to go out with me looking like this', then you'll feel down on yourself.

These feelings can then impact on our behaviour. For example, feeling negatively about our bodies can lead to behaviours aimed at altering appearance (e.g., excessive exercise, food restriction, checking our appearance over and over). It may also lead to avoidance behaviour (e.g., avoidance of social situations for fear of negative evaluation). When we start behaving in response to our negative body image, we often behave in ways that make us feel worse. The trick is to notice that you're feeling negative towards your body and having negative self-talk and decide to do something about it. This involves changing your behaviour in order to influence your beliefs and thoughts. The following chapter looks at how to change your behaviour to change your thoughts and feelings. First, here are a few activities to do.

ACTIVITIES

Ask yourself: 'What things do you do or avoid doing because of your body image? What do you do when you feel bad about your body?'

Think of examples in your own life that fit this ABC model and think about past events that may also have impacted on your thoughts and beliefs. For example, you might go to a party and feel that all the other women/men are more attractive than yourself, which activates the belief (I'm not attractive enough) which leads you to feel negative and perhaps you don't talk to others as much or you leave early.

Think back to the influences in your life both positive and negative that have assisted in forming your beliefs about your body and yourself. This is not about blaming others for our feelings or body image but about gaining insight into why we think and behave the way we do. Once we have the insight, we can more effectively work on changing the way we think and behave in order to feel better.

A

Antecedent or activating event

You see someone who you perceive is atractive or desirable walking past.

B

Belief or thought

You think 'I am so unattractive in comparison to them. I am sure everyone is looking at me and thinking how disgusting I look. If I only I could lose weight I'd be happy'.

C

Consequence, feeling and behaviour

You feel depressed and down on yourself. Your restrict what you eat that day and fit in an extra session at the gym which you don't enjoy.

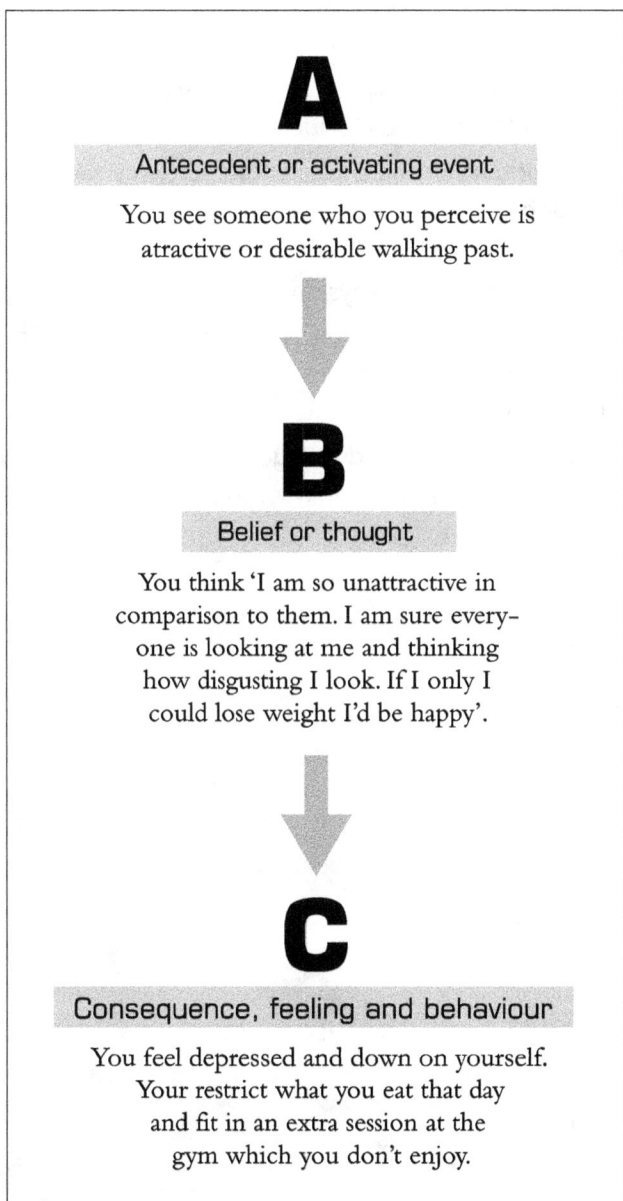

An example of the ABCs of body image can be seen in the figure above

CHAPTER SUMMARY

▌ Our experiences growing up, including our parents, peers, media as well as our genetics and personality, influence the development of our body image.

▌ The ABCs of body image tell us that it is the way we think about our body and appearance that needs changing in order to feel more positive.

▌ If we behave in positive ways, this also leads to feeling better.

▌ Identifying the current influences on our body image and identifying our own self-talk helps identify where and how we want to change.

▌ In order to change our body image, we first need to be aware of our own thinking, what we want to change, and then we can go about changing it.

Chapter 5

Changing your behaviour to change feelings

What makes me feel good about my body and self is getting up in the mornings and going for a walk. Getting out in the fresh air and getting my body moving gives me a great start to the day. I also know I've got my exercise out of the way for the day! When I start the day off with my walk I feel better and therefore am much more likely to continue with my health goals throughout the day.

Anthony, 55

Anthony struggled with obesity for 10 years. When he sought help he wasn't doing any physical activity at all and was binge eating every day. He was told if he didn't change his lifestyle he'd likely have a premature death. Many people like Anthony struggle with weight to the point it affects their physical and psychological health. The solution that people are given is often 'lose weight'. This is something people like Anthony have heard time and time again. As discussed in previous chapters, when our goal is to stop doing something, it is so much harder to achieve as the goal is seen as negative. When we turn the goal around to the positive, and in Anthony's case to feel healthier including to be able to walk more, people are much more likely to achieve it and stay motivated.

The first step in changing our body image is understanding how our behaviour influences our feelings. As we have already noted, we often think that we feel a certain way because of the situation or that events trigger certain feelings in us. But it's actually our own thinking and behaviour that triggers our feelings. For example, two people can be experiencing the same event but feel totally differently about it. Why? Because of the way they both interpret or think about the event. For example, have you ever noticed that at a party people appear to be experiencing it in different ways? Some are enjoying themselves, some are quiet and some look completely bored. They're all experiencing the same situation but everyone feels differently. This is due to what is going on in each person's head. Some may have just had an argument with someone and so are thinking negatively about that, some may be focusing on how much they enjoy party conversation and so feel good and others may be excited by the event and therefore feel high in spirits. Have you noticed that you yourself can sometimes be in the same situation and feel differently on different occasions? The situation is the same, but you feel differently. And this is due to your thoughts, what's going on in your head. So it makes sense that, if we could change what is going on in our heads, we can change the way we feel. Too often we hope the situation will change, like our boss or our partner behaving differently, but if we learn to think differently we will actually feel better about the situation. The following chapter looks at how we change our thinking. But first let's look at how our behaviour influences our feelings and how, if we change the way we behave, it will lead to more positive feelings.

Treat your body well

There is a strong link between the way we behave and treat our body and how we feel about it. Have you ever noticed that when you're not happy with your body you punish it through overeating or under-eating or missing out on social get togethers, wearing clothes that are unflattering or doing excessive exercise? And how does this make you feel? It makes you feel miserable usually.

We're punishing ourselves unnecessarily and it doesn't achieve anything but make us feel worse. Correct? Think about the last time you did something negative because you felt bad. Maybe this was drinking to excess because you'd experienced a break-up or a stressful event. Think about how it led you to feel worse and I bet it didn't solve the problem, right?

> *When I have a bad day, all I can think of is having a few beers and washing my sorrows away. Then the next day, the problems are there again.*
>
> *Roger, 45*

When we have stress and tension, we need constructive ways to handle or resolve it. There are many temporary measures such as eating and drinking that distract us, but they don't solve the problem and they don't really help in the long term. Exercise and healthy eating make us better able to cope with stress and keep our heads clear so we can better problem-solve. See Chapter 11 for general health tips including tips on managing stress and tension as well as dealing with anxiety and body distress in Chapter 6.

Imagine how you'd feel if you treated your body well. If you ate foods your body liked in moderation, you gave it plenty of water for hydration, exercised with friends, wore your favourite clothes, gave it plenty of rest including sleep and didn't work it too hard. You'd probably feel good. Think again about the last time you engaged in a positive behaviour and how it made you feel.

ACTIVITY

Ask yourself: 'What positive behaviour have I done recently and how did I feel during and after?'

When I feel a bit flat I have a glass of water or a piece of fruit and that helps clear my head.

Amanda, 60

Many people don't realise that in order to feel good about your body you have to treat it well. Our bodies are the only ones we have and, if we don't treat them well, no-one else will. Have a practice today doing something nice for your body and see how it makes you feel. For example, you might treat your body to something nice like a bath, walk or swim. Sometimes rating your mood out of 10 before and after you've engaged in an activity can help you work out what maximises your feel-good emotions.

Thank your body for all the things it does. Our bodies are amazing things. They help us walk, shop, relax, sleep, cuddle, talk, etc. We often take our bodies for granted and don't fully appreciate what they do for us.

Whenever I catch myself looking at my tummy and caesarean section scars with a less then positive thought, I say to myself that my tummy helped me bear my two beautiful children and that my scars are a sign of that.

Mandy, 38

Activity

Write down some of the things that you do that make you feel good. What are the positive behaviours you engage in regularly and rarely? Keep adding to your list and be prepared to do them when you catch yourself feeling a bit down. Even better, do them every day to prevent feeling down.

Think about the function of your body

Sometimes thinking about the function of your body can help you appreciate it more. I know this is hard especially if you're injured or unwell or you experience a lot of pain in your body. But thinking about each body part and what it helps you do can help you re-focus from what you don't like about the way your body looks to how your body parts serve a function and how they do it well. For example, from 'I don't like my big bottom' to 'My bottom helps me sit comfortably on a chair'; 'I have flabby arms' to 'my arms allow me to cuddle my family'; 'My chest is hairy and I don't like it' to 'My chest is hairy because of my genetics and race which makes me unique'. It's what we call in psychology a positive reframe where you take a negative statement and turn it into a positive. Have a practice now with a part of your body you often criticise and turn it around to a positive function. What positive behaviours can you now do to reinforce this to yourself?

> ### ACTIVITY
>
> Think of your body parts for their function — what do they allow you to do?

Do something with your body to feel better

Have you ever noticed how, when you feel down, doing something like calling a friend or leaving the house makes you feel better? There is a wealth of research looking at the doing part and how this makes us feel better. For example, did you know that doing something social improves your mood? That exercising actually assists depression? Why does doing things make us feel better? The reasons lie in the activation of the brain and release of feel good chemicals called endorphins. When our bodies are moving, the brain is more active which leads to an increase in mood due to neurochemical activity. As well, when our body is active, endorphins, or feel-good chemicals, are released by the brain.

So one of the ways to feel better about your body and yourself is to behave differently towards it. When we don't move our bodies, they can't feel energy or enthusiasm. Some ways to feel better about your body through doing include:

Being physically active — being active gets the blood pumping and also releases endorphins or the feel-good chemicals that lift our mood. Doing something with your body is also a great way to improve your body image. Focus on what you've done and what you've achieved rather than how far you might have to go if you have a fitness goal. Every step is a step closer.

Bask in the moment — happiness is a journey not a destination. So enjoy your journey towards your goals. Enjoy your exercise and fitness activity. Think about how good your body feels being active. Can you feel your muscles working? Turn the pain into a marker of achievement.

Make your skin feel nice — pampering your body, such as through touch and smell (wearing perfumes, moisturising our skin, shaving), revitalises the skin and body and makes us feel better. This is a very individual thing, though, so work out what suits you and your body. What smells do you like? What cloth feels nice against your body? Clean sheets when going to bed, for example, can feel really comfortable and nice against your skin, helping you sleep better.

Get enough sleep — sleep is necessary to revitalise the body and brain. See Chapter 11 on general health for more information on the benefits of sleep and sleep hygiene, and how you can get a better night's sleep.

Just try for the next week doing something every day to feel good and record how you feel before and after, like a little experiment. Give it a go for a few days so you can really test it.

Eating for emotional reasons or reasons other than hunger

Changing behaviour to feel better also involves changing our behaviour around food. For example, what would happen if you ate for your *body's* needs rather than *emotional* needs? People eat for all sorts of reasons other than being hungry. We can eat for emotional reasons such as being sad or upset, bored, happy, angry or anxious. Eating for these reasons often leads to negative feelings in the long run because we overeat and feel guilty or we think eating will make us feel better and it doesn't; it may just confirm our lack of control over eating or make us feel over full and lethargic and less like doing anything else. So next time we feel sad, bored, angry etc., try and do something more helpful. Ask yourself, 'How am I feeling and what will actually make me feel better, not just in the short term, but in the long term?' For example, if you feel sad, ask yourself what will help and comfort you. Do you need comfort from someone else — to talk to a friend?

The following chapter tackles the issue of anxiety and body behaviours including binge eating and how to increase your feelings of control. The chapter on eating disorders is also particularly useful for those trying to manage their eating.

Write a list of things you can do to respond to your emotions that will make you feel better. When I feel sad, lonely, tired, bored, angry, what can I do to feel better that will have a lasting effect?

Although not behaviours, positive affirmations are also another way to feel better about yourself. Telling yourself you're a good person and listing all your positives will help when you're feeling down. If you're feeling depressed, you may still feel down after reading your affirmations but you won't feel as bad as you did before. Request the help of those around you or pull out old cards or things you may have kept from others that give you compliments or make you feel good. We need to remind ourselves when we're feeling down of all the positive things that have happened in our life, the compliments, the praise, and those feel-good moments. Looking through photos, for example, can help remind ourselves of fun times we've had and significant people in our lives.

ACTIVITY

Write a list now of all your positive qualities. We've all got them. Think of the things you're good at, talents, what makes you a good friend, what makes you part of the community, your hobbies etc. Then ask someone else close to you, such as a friend or family member, to add to your list. You can keep adding to this list forever, adding more and more positive affirmations of who you are as a person and what makes you valuable.

CHAPTER SUMMARY

∎ Changing our behaviour (what we do) changes our feelings about our bodies and selves.

∎ Treating your body well will increase positive feelings.

∎ Find constructive helpful ways to deal with stress that have more than just a temporary effect.

∎ Eat foods for their function in your body.

∎ What behaviours can you increase to maximise feeling good?

∎ Treat your body well and you will feel more positive about it.

∎ Positive affirmations remind us about our body's value.

Chapter 6

Dealing with anxiety and body distress

I would spend all day thinking and worrying about the foods I ate and what they were doing to my body. If I ate a sweet for morning tea I'd spend the whole day thinking about how many calories it was, how I was going to work it off, and beating myself up for eating it. I couldn't focus on my work or people's conversations. I would say I felt distressed, my mind was fixated on these thoughts and I felt on edge.

Melanie, 37

This chapter continues looking at behaviour change but specifically in terms of reducing distress. The term distress is used to describe a negative experience in our bodies physiologically (such as a racing heart) and in our thinking which is often irrational or occurs without any realistic reason.

What behaviours can we change, stop or take up to feel better about our bodies and selves? Anxiety and stress are common feelings and can become distressing. Sometimes in order to reduce or eliminate this distress we engage in certain behaviours. These behaviours can be both helpful or a hindrance. Here we're going to look at balancing out our behaviours to feel less distressed. People often say to me that they want to stop feeling stressed. It's important to realise that stress doesn't have to always be negative. A little bit of stress is actually helpful. Getting a little stressed before a presentation, for example, helps us perform better. A little stress can also help us get things done. Ever studied super hard the day before an exam or powered through a task because the stress has increased your motivation? What about when you're in danger and the stress response has helped you escape? Stress is important for general functioning. If we had no stress we'd be dead. Our body would stop functioning. It is stress that keeps our heart pumping, our brain thinking, our body working. What is not good stress is too much of it — where we become overwhelmed by the symptoms of stress such as racing thoughts, agitation, feelings of panic, desire to run away when nothing is actually threatening us but we *perceive* that something is.

So when people talk about wanting to reduce their stress, they mean reducing feelings of stress when they need and want to feel calm. Reducing stress is about two things: one, calming down your body's physiological arousal (heart rate, sweating, temperature, muscle tension); and two, calming your thinking down. These two things will lead you to feel more relaxed. It is almost impossible to feel stressed if your body is calm and we can calm our bodies in any way that lowers our heart rate and physiological arousal. Some people use structured ways such as relaxation techniques and others may use self-soothing statements and methods to reduce thinking and the body's own processing.

There are many behaviours such as drinking or eating that we do over and over again, thinking they will make us feel better. Sometimes they do but this is usually only temporary. For example, if you've broken up with someone, you may want to have a few drinks, thinking it will make you feel better. Perhaps numbing the pain (and our consciousness) works in the short term but as soon as the alcohol wears off the problem is still there. We haven't solved it through this behaviour. Let's call behaviour that doesn't solve the problem 'negative behaviour' and ask yourself, 'What could I do instead that would make me feel better in a way that has a more lasting effect or doesn't also have negative consequences such as a hangover?' For example, often talking to someone, treating your body well, or getting some exercise for stress relief has a more lasting and positive effect.

<hr>

ACTIVITY

Have a think now about what it is that you do that makes you feel better more than just momentarily and doesn't have negative consequences. Write these things down and practice doing them as coping strategies.

Quick relief techniques to manage anxiety

There are some situations that cause us to feel anxious and self-conscious about our bodies and if we can't prepare ahead of time for these we need what psychologists call 'quick relief' strategies or techniques for managing our anxiety.

Although we may not be able to completely eradicate our anxiety, we can certainly reduce it or make it more manageable. Some quick relief techniques include:

Calming statements: these are statements we can make to ourselves that are reassuring, such as 'I'll be ok' or 'I can do this'. What statements work for you? Think back to previous occasions where you've felt anxious and what you have told yourself. If you're feeling self-conscious, perhaps you could tell yourself, 'No-one is looking at me', or repeating the word 'calm' to yourself. Try to think of situations you've been in where you've coped. Use these examples to help sooth your thoughts. You may ask your partner or a friend to help remind you of your calming statements or reassuring statements that you'll cope in this situation.

Breathing: slowing down your breathing as much as possible, getting the same amount of air in as out can help calm your body physiologically. As well, focusing on your breathing helps you distract yourself and calms your thinking down. Try breathing in for 4 seconds, hold for 2, out for 4, and repeating your calming statements. Do this for at least two minutes or until you feel calmer. It is hard to panic and get anxious when your breathing is controlled. Practice this in non-anxious situations so that when you're in an anxious situation you can turn it on automatically. The trick is to make your breathing slow and controlled and to focus only on it.

Being mindful: this involves trying to focus on what you're doing, your surrounds and taking your attention off yourself. For example, if you're feeling anxious at a party, focus on what the other person is saying rather than how you're feeling. If you're at the swimming pool in your swimmers and you start to feel uncomfortable or worried others are looking at you, focus on looking at others, the water, feeling the heat or the grass where you're sitting. Focus on what you are doing, seeing, hearing, smelling, tasting, rather than the negative or anxious thoughts floating around in your head. You are focusing on the present rather than the anxious thoughts in your head; this is part of mindfulness. Sometimes it can help to focus on the things you can hear, see, feel, smell and taste rather than being overwhelmed by the thoughts in your head. This is a particularly useful technique for those of us trying to pay more attention to what we're eating. If we're trying to stop eating so quickly as is the case in binge eating, slowing it down and focusing on the act of eating, the smell, taste, texture, can help to stop binge eating through drawing our attention to what we're doing. Try eating a meal over 20 minutes. This requires us to eat slowly, with a knife and fork and focus purely on the act of eating and how it feels, tastes, smells, looks, sounds. Cut out other distractions such as television and just focus on the task at hand. This *mindfulness eating approach* will help yous enjoy your food more, give your stomach time to tell your brain it's full by slowing down your eating and make you more conscious of what you're putting in your mouth, as one of the problems with binge eating is eating mindlessly, without consciousness.

*At the end of the day I look forward to what I call my mindful-
ness time. I set aside 10 minutes every afternoon to sitting outside
in my yard and I think about what I can see in the garden, what
I can hear, what I can feel which is often the cool breeze on my
face, what I can smell in the garden and what I can touch. Doing
this every day helps me keep my focus and stop the busyness of
the day getting ahead of me.*

Sonia, 65.

ACTIVITY

Try this activity now to become more in the moment. When
we're in the moment, it's much harder to be anxious and stressed
because we're focusing on the here and now rather than the
stresses of the past or future. Try just sitting for 5 minutes and
becoming aware of five things that you can see, five things you
can hear, five things you can touch (i.e., the chair you're sitting
on, your clothes on your skin, your hair on your shoulders), and
what you can smell (i.e., your body lotion, the room, food, fresh
air) and possibly taste (i.e., toothpaste, what you've just eaten).
This mindfulness activity helps to ground you in the present. Use
it when you feel stressed or overwhelmed by things to quickly
pull you into the present.

Challenging your thinking and dealing with anxious situations and distress

This is discussed in more detail in the next chapter. When you're
feeling self-conscious, challenging your thoughts can also work
here, looking for the evidence against your irrational and/or distressing thinking. So if you're worried everyone is looking at
you, look for the evidence for and against; you might find that,
mostly, no-one is looking at you. If you are in a highly feared situation you may need to break it down and take it in smaller

steps. See Chapter 8 for devising a fear hierarchy. Setting up rewards for getting through an anxiety-provoking situation may also be helpful and encouraging for you. Turn to Chapter 14 for more assistance with this.

Some preventative strategies for anxiety management and reducing your distress involve preparing your body and mind ahead of time. If you know you're going to be anxious in a situation that is ahead of you, prepare for it. Work on reducing your anxiety leading up to the situation. What can you do? What can you say to yourself that will help? This is a great time to practice challenging your negative self-defeating thoughts. Ask yourself, 'What am I worried about?', and then, 'Is this realistic or an irrational fear? How likely is it that this worry will actually happen? What's the evidence for and against?' Then, 'How can I replace this thought with a more southing, relaxing, realistic and helpful thought?'

Many people find regular relaxation assists them to cope with anxiety. For some, relaxation will be in the form of sitting quietly, going for a walk, listening to calming music and for some it will be progressive muscle relaxation. Relaxation involves reducing the heart rate as well as calming our thoughts. Let's look at the benefits of relaxation now, and specifically a type of relaxation called *progressive muscle relaxation*.

Relaxation to manage anxiety

One of the effects of having a negative body image is increased anxiety. Anxiety can arise in many different situations for people with a negative body image, such as catching your reflection in the mirror, being at the gym and noticing someone looking at you, or trying on clothes. Social situations may also lead to increased anxiety and to feeling self-conscious. One common technique used to treat anxiety is relaxation. Relaxation involves trying to focus your attention on soothing thoughts and decreasing tension in the body. There are lots of different ways people relax including deep breathing, going somewhere soothing such as a beach, or reading a book. *Progressive muscle relaxation* is one psychological technique for working towards managing your anxiety. A script is outlined below — you may prefer your own script or method of relaxation, but try this one. It usually takes people a few practices to master it and then you can call upon it when needed. The following activity will take about 20 minutes but you can speed it up or slow it down depending on how long you spend getting comfortable at the start and enjoying the relaxation at the end. Be careful not to tense each muscle too much or you main strain a muscle. Also, be careful when tensing your back and neck. Do it gently at first so as not to pull a muscle. If you feel a spasm or pain, stop, stretch, and try and relax the muscle. If you are pregnant or have back injuries, do not tense these areas as you may cause yourself injury.

Progressive muscle relaxation script

Find a quiet space and lie down on a bed or floor or sit comfort-ably and close your eyes. Take a minute to settle yourself and get comfortable. Try and focus on how comfortable it feels having your eyes closed, enjoying the quiet and feeling relaxed. Keep your breathing slow and regular, about four breaths in and two hold, four out. Some people like to say something to themselves like the word 'calm' as they relax each part, to help them get further into the relaxation.

You're now going to go through each major muscle in your body and feeling the difference between tension and relaxation. We're going to start with your toes and feet. I want you to point your toes and feet and hold this position for a few seconds. Focus on the tightness in your toes, feet and ankles. After a few seconds release this tension, feeling all the stress go out of your toes, feet and ankles and rest your feet on the floor or bed. Wriggle your toes and feel the difference between tension and relaxation.

Next I want you to focus on your legs — one way to tense your legs is to flex your feet upright and lengthen-out your legs, feeling a slight pull. Feel this tension for a few seconds and then release, letting your legs flop down onto the bed or floor. Feel the difference between tension and relaxation in your legs.

Wait a few seconds and focus on the relaxation through your legs, feet and toes before moving on to your buttocks. Now focus on tensing your buttocks. You can do this by squeezing your cheeks together tightly and feeling the tension throughout your buttocks. Hold this tension for a few seconds and then let it go slowly, feeling all the tension drift out of your buttocks. Feel the relaxation through your buttocks, legs, ankles, feet and toes.

Next, focus on your back. You can feel the tension in your back by arching it and trying to squeeze your shoulder blades together. Hold this tension for a few seconds, really focusing on the tension in your lower and upper back. Hold the tension and then let it go and relax. Feel all the tension drift out of your lower and upper back, out of your shoulder blades. Just relax on the chair or bed and feel the relaxation in your back, buttocks, legs, feet and toes.

The next body part is your shoulders. You can tense your shoulders by shrugging them and bringing them up to your ears and holding them there for a few seconds. Feel the tension in your shoulders and then let go. Feel all the tension wash out of your shoulders, down your back, past your buttocks, down your legs, through your ankles and out of your toes.

Next you're going to focus on your arms and wrists. Stretch out your arms in front of you as far as they will go and hold this tension. Hold it for a few seconds and then let it go. Feel all the tension drop out of your arms as you flop your arms beside you. Now you're going to focus on your fingers. Span your fingers wide as far apart as they will go and hold. Hold this tension in your fingers and then let it go. Relax your fingers, your wrists, your arms and feel all of the tension going out of our arms, wrists and fingers. Feel the relaxation in your shoulders, your back, your buttocks, your legs, your ankles, your feet and your toes. All the tension is leaving your body.

Next you're going to focus on your neck. Gently try to touch your left ear to your left shoulder, stretching out the right side of your neck. Hold this for a few seconds and then bring your head up to the centre and stretch it to the other side, hold it there for a few seconds and then move it back to the centre. Feel all of the tension release on both the left and right sides of your neck. Now stretch your head backwards in order to stretch the front of your neck. Feel the tension in the front of your neck and then slowly release your head back to the centre again. Now move your head trying to touch your chin to your chest to stretch the back of your neck. Hold this for a few seconds and then slowly release. You might like to move your head gently to relax it further. Focus on how relaxed your neck feels, the relaxation in your shoulders, no tension in your back or buttocks, no tension in your legs or ankles and no tension in your feet and toes. Take a few seconds to focus on each of these parts and how relaxed you feel.

Lastly we're going to focus on relaxing the face. First you're going to relax your forehead. You can do this by frowning as hard as you can. Hold this frown for a few seconds and then let it go. Feel the smoothness of your forehead. Now to your eyes: with your eyes shut, squeeze them shut for a few seconds. Now slowly relax your eyes. Keep them shut but focus on how much more relaxed they feel, how relaxed your brow feels. Focus on the relaxation in your face. Now to your mouth and cheeks: bite down on your teeth whilst smiling to feel the tension in your mouth and cheeks. Do this for a few seconds and then let go. Focus on how relaxed your face feels, your neck feels, your back, your buttocks, your legs, ankles, feet and toes. Focus on this for a few seconds.

Now scan your body for any last bit of tension. Wherever there is tension, tense that part of your body for a few seconds and then release it, feeling the tension go from your whole body.

Now just sit or lie for a few minutes enjoying your relaxation. Focus on each body part and how relaxed it feels; how nice each part feels.

When you're ready, slowly become aware of the room you're in and open your eyes. Stay lying down or sitting for a little longer to orientate yourself to the room before getting up. When you get up, get up slowly, have a drink of water as sometimes relaxation can dehydrate you, and go about your day feeling more relaxed and calm.

Throughout the day, when you feel a muscle getting tense you can tense this muscle as you did here and let the tension go, focusing on the relaxation of that body part.

You may like to tape yourself reading this script so you can play it back to yourself to use every day or when needed.

Summary on changing behaviour to change thinking and feeling

Let's take this opportunity to summarise where we're up to. Changing thinking and feeling also involves changing the way we behave. If we behave in a way that supports a positive thought, it is much harder to feel unhappy or distressed about our appearance. For example, if we get out of the house when we least feel like it, we start thinking more clearly and feel more energised and thus more positive about our body and self. Have you ever noticed that when you feel down or depressed you start to behave in ways that maintain this feeling or make it worse? How many of us have stayed in bed when we felt unhappy or sat on the couch and ate, feeling more and more miserable? We need to do the opposite even though we may not like it. If when we're feeling miserable we get up and go for a walk or go and see a friend we do feel better. Try it if you haven't already, and test out the theory. Do I feel better when I'm more active? Do I feel better when I socialise more? Do I feel better when I treat my body to pampering?

CHAPTER SUMMARY

▌ Stress can be helpful in moderation to help motivate us to get things done or help us perform better or when we're excited.

▌ Stress is negative when it impacts on our bodies, health and mind in ways that make us feel overwhelmed, tense and unwell.

▌ Stress reduction involves reducing the body's arousal and calming our thoughts.

▌ There are many things we do that relieve stress in the short term such as drugs and alcohol but have harmful effects in the long term.

▌ Quick relief techniques can be used anywhere at any time to manage stress.

▌ Trying to be in the moment and focusing on what's going on around you rather than what's in your head can help give you calm.

▌ Take time to just be in the moment and try and focus on the one task — eating, relaxing, etc.

▌ Relaxation is a great tool for long-term anxiety control. You need to practice it every day though.

Chapter 7

Changing the way you think to change the way you feel

I used to tell myself I was stupid or an idiot if I made a mistake like forgetting to do something. This made me feel worse and I'd really be down on myself. Everyone makes mistakes and making a mistake doesn't make me flawed as a person. All I can do is learn and move forward. Having a more balanced thinking style helps me keep things in perspective and stops me beating myself up.

Peter, 45

Remember in Chapter 4 how we talked about the key to changing the way we feel is to change the way we think or our beliefs about our physical appearance? This is the B (beliefs) out of our ABC model. Changing the way we think about our bodies and selves is challenging. Often we've been thinking the same way about our bodies for a long time and we've taught ourselves to automatically think negatively. Remember also in Chapter 4 how we talked about the influences on our body image? These have helped form our beliefs and our current influences — such a media and the society we live in — often maintain these beliefs.

Here you're going to try and think more positively about your body and yourself. It may not be possible to like everything or be 100% happy with your body but you can certainly improve the way you think about your body and reduce the distress you may feel as a result of the way you're thinking.

Changing thinking requires a conscious effort to think differently. Firstly, we have to become aware of the way we think in order to change it. You might like to write down ways you catch yourself thinking about your body. For example, 'What do I say to myself when someone gives me a compliment? What do I say when I look in the mirror?'

There are behaviours we have that maintain our negative thinking about our bodies, and these include avoiding situations where we feel uncomfortable with our bodies, repeatedly checking our bodies for the perceived defect or the parts we don't like, as well as looking for evidence that convinces us our body isn't right or is ugly. Our attention to negative reinforcement of our negative beliefs about our bodies is heightened. So part of overcoming body image distress and dissatisfaction is to stop doing these things. We talked in the previous chapters about stopping our ritualistic behaviours and stopping avoiding situations. Here we'll learn how to stop looking for evidence that supports a negative body image and instead challenge our beliefs about our bodies and start looking for more balanced evidence that counters our negative beliefs and possibly replaces them with more helpful and more positive beliefs. Firstly, we'll learn about challenging negative thinking and how to reduce if not stop that inner critique making us feel bad about our bodies. This will involve looking at typical cognitive or thinking errors people make and then how we change our beliefs.

Changing our beliefs is not an easy task as we've often been thinking this way for a long time. So we need to be willing to look for alternative beliefs and be willing to see that there is another side to our thinking and that there is evidence that supports a more positive body image. Here, you need to focus on being optimistic. It may help in this section to think if I was doing this with my best friend what would I say. Often if we look at ourselves and our thoughts from an outsider's perspective it can be easier to challenge our negative thinking.

The first step to challenging our negative thinking and beliefs about our bodies is to become aware of our thinking. Often the thoughts go through our heads without us being aware of them. So first we need to draw our attention to them so we can work on replacing them with more helpful and balanced thoughts.

Step 1: Be aware of your thinking

Write down your typical thoughts about your appearance. What thoughts or beliefs go through your head when you think about your appearance? What things trigger these thoughts? Once we know how we're thinking, we're better able to change it. The other typical thing that occurs with our thinking is that we make assumptions about our appearance or the appearance of others. For example, 'If I was thin, I'd have more success at meeting men; 'if my eyes weren't so close together I'd get a girlfriend'; 'that person is overweight and therefore is ugly'. Have a think about the assumptions you make about yourself as these hold us back for feeling positive about our appearance.

Also, what assumptions do you make about others? For example, what assumptions do you have about people you perceive are attractive? Some common assumptions we make about those who are attractive are that they are lucky or can get anything they want. But these are just assumptions — they're not based on fact. So I ask you to think about the assumptions you make about others or yourself and ask what's the evidence for this belief.

ACTIVITY

Write down what your thoughts are about your appearance. What assumptions do you make about how you and others look and what this means? Do these assumptions help or hinder you achieving a positive body image?

Step 2: Look for the evidence for and against this thought

One way we can change our thinking is to do what psychologists call *examining the evidence*. This means, rather than simply accepting the beliefs you have, actually ask yourself, 'What's the evidence for this belief?' or 'Why do I think this is true?' Often there are beliefs we have that have no evidence to support them or some evidence for and against. The question then is, if there is no evidence, why am I holding onto this belief? Perhaps I need to re-evaluate my belief and even discard it.

Changing thinking is all about seeing things more realistically. So, where you have a particular thought that might be distressing to you, challenge the evidence for it and try and replace it with a more realistic and even helpful thought. For example, if you believe thin people have it all, ask yourself, 'What is the evidence for this?' Look at both sides of the argument. You probably know of some thin people who have a lot of desirable things but also many people who are not thin who have desirable things. There are also probably a lot of thin people who have very little. Try to have a more realistic and helpful thought — something like 'Thin people don't have it all' or 'Having it all is not dependent on your body size'. This more realistic way of seeing things will go a long way, for example, in making you feel better about your size and shape.

So write down now some of the common assumptions you've made about people's appearance and the reality of these assumptions. Look at how you can replace these assumptions with more helpful ways of thinking.

Remember from Chapter 4 that our thoughts are often automatic and pop into our head without us consciously being aware of them sometimes. So be on the lookout for noticing where you engage in negative thinking or making appearance assumptions and deliberately try and challenge the way you think rather than just accepting it.

*I always thought beautiful people have it all. If only I was beau-
tiful I'd have it all too, or at least my life would be better than I
perceived it to be. Through the help of a psychologist, I learnt
how to challenge this appearance assumption I had. I started to
think of all the people I knew of varying shapes and size and
degrees of 'idealised' attractiveness I had in my head and the
things I loved about them which weren't related to how they
looked at all. I thought, if I can do this with other people, why
can't I do this for myself?*

Trisha, 55

Changing our beliefs about appearance

It's been identified that past influences impact on the development
of body image, but the question still remains, how is this so? Past
experiences can influence our thoughts, as they lead to the development of certain learnt beliefs about the meaning of appearance in
life. Such beliefs influence and guide the kinds of things that we pay
attention to, how we think about life events and about ourselves.
These beliefs become so ingrained that we take them as truth. For
example, if we are constantly bombarded with obesity warnings in
the media, we learn that fat is bad. But in reality we need some
body fat in order to fuel our body and brain. We also need body fat
to keep warm, for pregnancy, to have something comfortable to sit
on, among other reasons. But this is an appearance belief we've
developed, so when we see someone in the shopping centre who is
obese and is eating takeaway we think, 'No wonder they look that
way, they're eating bad foods'. But there could be a million other
explanations for their weight, such as genetics, health reasons etc.

There are many different experiences in our lives that can lead
to the development of appearance assumptions. One major step
towards improving body image is arguing with these appearance
assumptions that we have developed over time. Which ones do you
have? Identify these and work on challenging through examining
the evidence for the belief and disputing the evidence. This can also
involve rules that we've established for ourselves but not for others,

such as 'It's ok for others to look any way they want to, but not for me'. Challenge this by asking yourself where this rule comes from and is it useful to have this rule.

Challenging negative thoughts and beliefs and replacing them with more helpful thoughts will lead us to feel better about our bodies and selves. Also, replacing appearance rules and assumptions with more balanced thinking will help. Once we're aware of our negative unhelpful thinking, we can decide to change.

Ask yourself, 'What would it be like if I saw my body more positively? What would I say? How would I act? How would I know I was thinking more positively?' Write down the thoughts you have and some of the common themes. Am I always comparing myself to others? Do I always look for the bad? Do I generalise from one experience? Psychologists call certain ways of negatively thinking 'cognitive errors' in thinking — ways we think that maintain bad feelings; for example, over-generalising. Let's now look at identifying our thinking errors.

Step 3: Identifying your thinking errors

We all make errors in our thinking including making assumptions about people's looks and thinking in absolute terms without considering alternatives or checking for the accuracy of our beliefs. There are some common ways of thinking that people have which are actually incorrect. If we can identify our incorrect thinking and challenge it to become more balanced, it will help us improve our body image and feelings about ourselves.

Go through the following common thinking errors, identify which ones apply to you and, like you did in the previous section, question this thinking and make it a more balanced thought and belief.

Some of the common errors in thinking are:

Comparing ourselves to unrealistic standards of 'beauty' or manliness for men — constantly comparing yourself to models or celebrities or others who we think have the bodies we want. Constantly comparing ourselves to others can lead to feelings of negativity towards our own bodies, particularly when we compare ourselves to celebrities or unrealistic images in the media including magazines.

All or nothing thinking where we're all good or all bad — we're either being healthy or we're not, rather than a balance. For example, how many of us have been 'dieting' and going along really well until we have something on our 'non-diet food' list only to tell ourselves we've blown our diet and so cease because we've been 'bad'? We need to learn about balance — we can't be 'good' all the time. We also have slip-ups but these don't have to become relapses. This often offers when we're working towards our goals. If we keep moving forward we're okay but as soon as we hit a tricky point or stumble we throw it all in and quit. This is an error in thinking. Rather, if we expect slip-ups and are willing to use them as learning experiences and not over-exaggerate them, we're much more likely to feel good and keep working towards our goals. This cognitive error also occurs in our 'food rules'. The rules we might have set for ourselves around what we can and can't eat or good foods vs bad foods. Thinking about food in absolute terms sets us up to fail as, if we eat something from the 'bad' food list, we feel guilty and negative about ourselves. It can sabotage our attempts at being healthy and happy. Have a think about some of the food rules you might have and if they are realistic and valid and whether there is a more balanced approach that allows for mistakes and variety. What other absolute rules do you have? Perhaps around exercise? Consider challenging absolute rules as they don't allow for variability and change but rather lead to stress, distress and dysfunction.

Selectively attending to certain body parts we don't like and exaggerating their negative impact. For example, 'I hate my thighs, therefore I'm ugly'. We might prefer parts of our bodies to be different but that doesn't make them ugly and it doesn't have to ruin the way we think about ourselves. Try and focus rather on what you like about your body or the function of those body parts rather than their faults.

Scapegoating — where we believe our physical appearance is directly responsible for our success or otherwise in life, the reason why we have or don't have certain things. Rather, we can determine our own destiny, not our physical appearance.

Mind-reading — where we make assumptions about what other people think about our appearance and us as people. For example, we might make the assumptions that everyone in the shopping centre is looking at us and evaluating our appearance badly. Ask yourself, what is the evidence for this? How do you know that? Question whether this is an assumption you're making rather than it actually being real. You might like to test it and look at what others are looking at.

Fortune telling — where we believe, because of our appearance, our destiny as a person is determined. For example, 'Because I was fat at school I won't ever find a partner who likes me'. Question this: is this actually true? What's the evidence for and against and what's a more balanced way of thinking?

Being bound by your looks or weight— where what we do is dominated by how we feel about our body. Where we think we can or can't do things because of the way we perceive we look. For example, 'I can't go out and socialise until I lose weight', or 'I can't ask that girl out until my muscles are just right'. If we waited until everything in our life was perfect we'd never do anything.

There are many, many more errors in thinking we do that lead us to feel unhappy with our bodies and selves. What ones do you have?

To summarise, it's important to identify thoughts and beliefs that are holding us back from enjoying life.

Step 4: Challenge your thinking errors.
What do I do once I've noticed the errors?

Once you've identified the errors you make, now you can start to challenge and change them. Ask yourself questions such as, 'What is the evidence for this thought? If I maintain this thought, how will I feel?' Be curious: 'What would happen if I thought differently? How would I feel if I thought my looks were ok, and that I didn't need to look perfect in order to socialise?'

Notice the effects of thinking differently and practice it — practice, practice, practice. Challenge negative thoughts to test them. Are they actually true or have you just convinced yourself that they're true?

ACTIVITY

With the following section, write down whether any of these fit for you and catch yourself doing it. Next, practice stopping this way of thinking through challenging it.

- If you over-generalise, ask, 'Is this the case in all situations?'
- If you constantly compare yourself to others, ask, 'Is this relevant to me?'
- If you constantly generalise from one bad situation, ask, 'Is this relevant to me now?

Catch yourself feeling bad about your body and ask yourself, 'What am I thinking? Is this true or an error in my thinking? How can I replace this thinking with something more helpful so I feel better?' Do something to make you feel good — something active that forces you to behave differently to feel better.'

Putting it all together

So now let's add to our ABC model where you thought about events that may have triggered or activated thoughts about your appearance. Then you thought about your beliefs, then the behavioural and feeling consequences of them. It is our thoughts that lead us to feel the way we do.

So how do we change our thinking, then, to feel better and more positive? How do we change a negative thought into a positive one? There are several ways to do this. One way is to dispute your thoughts by asking yourself how realistic are your thoughts? Once we can dispute our thoughts, we can correct them. This correction, with practice, should lead to feeling and behaving more positively. Let's look at an example.

You see your friend who you think is attractive. This is the activating or antecedent event. You immediately think, 'I am unattractive in comparison to them, I am ugly in comparison'. This is the thought or belief. As a consequence you feel down and bad about yourself and may decide to go home early because you're not feeling good about yourself and eat foods that make you feel worse about yourself. This consequence is in your feelings and behaviour.

What would happen if you disputed the thought 'I'm unattractive in comparison to my friend'? What if you asked yourself, 'What's the evidence for this thought? What are the facts?' Perhaps you might say, 'My friend is attractive, but that doesn't mean I'm unattractive in comparison. We're different and not comparable. What comments has my friend given me? Perhaps they've commented on how good it is to see me so I should focus on that rather than my appearance.'

This challenging of your thinking and being more realistic would lead you to focus on your friend rather than your appearance, therefore increasing your enjoyment of your time with them. You're more likely to enjoy your day and not go home early or sabotage your health goals.

Everyone goes through similar experiences day to day, but it is our interpretation of these experiences that influences how we feel. It takes practice to challenge the way we think and change automatic negative thinking. Every day, when you catch yourself thinking a particularly negative way, question your thinking, challenge it, look for the alternative evidence and try and re-focus your attention to the positive or at least a more balanced way of thinking.

Here's another example where we may have received some criticism. It's natural when we receive criticism to not feel very good about it but it's our choice as to how much we let this criticism affect us. For example, often we hold onto negative comments about our appearance (or quality, talent, character, etc.) that we've received in the past. When this past criticism is interfering with our present, we need to ask ourselves a few questions: How relevant is this criticism to us now? Do I want this criticism to continue to pull me down? What's a more balanced way of considering this criticism so it doesn't bother me so much?

ACTIVITY

Have a go now at a situation you've caught yourself in recently and dispute your thoughts and re-evaluate the situation. Then how do you feel different?

On top of challenging our negative body image, we also need to focus on promoting a positive body image and sense of self. One way to do this is to focus on the things you like about yourself and the things you're good at or interested in. You keep repeating these to yourself until they become your automatic way of thinking rather than the negative. Chapter 12 is dedicated to feeling good about your whole self, not just your body image. Read this and work on feeling better about the whole you. As well, the following tips on saying positive things to your body and self, and learning to accept compliments, can help improve your body image and overall wellbeing.

Positive affirmations for our whole self

We all have talents and qualities that make us special and unique as people. There is something good in everyone and sometimes we need to remind ourselves of this. Have a go now listing 10 things you like about yourself such as qualities of your personality, things you're good at, positive ways your treat others, or any aspect of yourself. These can be large or small.

It's also important, in liking ourselves as a whole, that we focus on the positive elements of our appearance, because we should love the skin we're in as well as what's inside of it. If you have difficulty listing what you like about your appearance — and it can be anything from your eyes, lips, hair, toes — try thinking about what a close friend might say about what they like about your appearance or compliments you've received.

Accepting compliments

On top of challenging the way we know we think about our bodies and our attitude towards them, in order to feel good about our bodies it's also important to be on the lookout for collecting the evidence that supports a positive body image. One way to do this is to collect compliments from others. Others are a great source of self-esteem building. So next time someone offers you a compliment about your appearance, accept it graciously and take it on board as evidence supporting a positive body image. Seeing ourselves through the eyes of others can often make us feel much more positive, as others have a much less biased opinion of us and they don't have all the same filters of influence we have towards our own bodies. Think about past compliments you've received also. These can be comments, smiles, gestures, or anything that gives you positive feedback.

CHAPTER SUMMARY

▮ Separate thoughts from feelings. The more we understand what goes on in our own head the more able we are to challenge and stop negative thinking.

▮ Don't just accept thoughts. Examine the evidence for them and come up with more balanced ways of thinking.

▮ Identify your errors in thinking that lead you to feel bad about yourself.

▮ Challenge your errors in thinking to be more balanced and positive.

▮ Make positives affirmations of yourself.

▮ Learn to accept compliments.

Chapter 8

Stopping ritualistic body behaviours and eliminating fears

I used to fear going out to dinner with friends. I obsessed over what I'd have to eat, what the quantity would be, what people would think about my eating, what others would order. I used to get so worked up I'd often be unable to go. I finally taught myself balanced thinking and talking myself down from totally irrational thoughts and faced my fears over eating what I thought were 'bad' foods. These are my friends, it's one event and I will enjoy it once I relax. I really examined my rules around eating and stopped focusing on myself and just enjoyed others' company.

Sally, 24.

All of us have habits or things that we do over and over to try and make ourselves feel better even though they may not be good for us. For example, we might overeat when we're unhappy or have to go to the gym every day even if we are injured to feel good and feel anxious if we don't. It's hard to stop doing certain behaviours even though we know they're not good for us. This chapter will help you erase the rituals or behaviours that you have and replace them with more adaptive and helpful ways of behaving. As well, this chapter looks at being assertive, especially around appearance comments you may receive from others.

The reasons for stopping such behaviours lies in the distress they cause us and the interference they have in our lives. For example, there's nothing wrong with going to a particular class at the gym five times a week and looking forward to this and enjoying it. But it becomes a problem if we feel compelled to go despite having something else important to do or where if we don't go we feel highly distressed and agitated. It's also a problem if this behaviour causes our body to became overtired or injured. Indicators such as family, friends or colleagues making comments or questioning why we do something can be indicators that our behaviour is obsessive. Also, where we think about something a lot and feel anxious until we've completed it. This can be seen in anxiety conditions such as Obsessive Compulsive Disorder where the person feels compelled to do something such as checking locks over and over to reduce their anxiety. It can also be seen in alcoholism where a person feels anxious until they've had a few drinks. It is also common when we have concerns with our weight or shape where we must exercise every day, otherwise we feel depressed or anxious, or where we mustn't eat certain foods or we fear we'll gain weight, or continuous thought processes like calorie counting.

This obsessive behaviour stops us enjoying life and relaxing because we feel compelled to do something. Have a think about whether there are any behaviours you may engage in that you would qualify as obsessive. Are there any mental processes that you do that are obsessive? If there are, ask yourself how you would feel if you weren't compelled to do them. More relaxed? Less anxious? In a better mood? If so, have a think about how you could slowly reduce this behaviour with the aim of feeling better. Use some of the techniques you've read about in earlier chapters and remember to start gradually moving through to harder steps as you master the easier ones.

What's wrong with doing things that reduce our anxiety? There's a difference between relaxation and compulsive behaviour. When we get a particular thought that goes over and over in our heads until we've done something about it, this is called an obsessive thought. It is following through with this thought that is the compulsive behaviour — behaviour you have to do to eliminate the obsession. People can do this with many things such as obsessively thinking about germs and therefore needing to wash hands over and over again to make the thought go away. Unfortunately, what happens when we carry out the behaviour is that it strengthens the obsession, making it more likely that this obsession will continue. This can occur with weight and shape also, where we might become obsessed with weighing ourselves, for example. We get the obsessive thought that we must weigh ourselves and we feel anxious until we've gone and checked. But unfortunately the checking doesn't always make us feel better. We can feel worse if the number isn't 'right' or feel the need to keep checking throughout the day to ensure the number doesn't change. This leads to a vicious cycle where we become dominated by the number on the scales. Let's now turn to looking at one form of ritualistic behaviour called checking and how to eliminate it.

How do I eliminate checking behaviour?

When we're trying to eliminate checking behaviour, we have to be prepared to sit with the uncomfortable feeling and desire to check. This often involves feeling high anxiety or being uncomfortable until it passes. This is where your relaxation techniques will be highly beneficial to distract you from checking and try and keep you calm. It will take a while and you need to keep practicing and stopping yourself checking. Eventually the urge will pass. The more you don't engage in the behaviour, the weaker the link gets between the obsessive thought and the behaviour, eventually eliminating it.

Using your cognitive strategies will also work well here, where you use calming statements and sayings to help calm you down and stop disputing your thoughts, particularly those that may sabotage your attempts such as 'just one last time'.

When we're trying to eliminate a compulsive behaviour we may need to do things to minimise the chances of us carrying out the activity, such as throwing away the scales, eliminating certain foods or doing things which mean we can't carry out the behaviour. Also, use the help of those around you so that you're more likely to be successful in your attempts at eliminating your actions.

Expect it to take time — if it's a behaviour you've been doing for a few years it will take some weeks or months to eliminate completely.

Activity

Write down the things you do that you would consider to be obsessive or excessive. These are often thing we feel compelled to do and feel very anxious about until we've done them. Then ask yourself, 'Does doing this activity actually make me feel better or does it feed my anxiety? What do I need to help me at this time?' To summarise:

- What is the behaviour I want to stop or reduce? (identify it clearly)
- How will I know if this behaviour is reduce or stopped? (make it measurable)
- What will help me to reduce or stop this behaviour (what coping tools will I use, what cognitive and behavioural strategies will I use, who will help me)?
- How will I reward myself for successfully reducing this behaviour?

Reminder of activities to keep doing

- Keep practicing relaxation and disputing automatic thoughts.
- Work on your healthy lifestyle change (turn to Chapter 11) — you may like to add physical exercise or nutrition goals to make you feel better in yourself (remember, it's not about looks).
- For parents, work on improving the family's healthy lifestyle.

- If you can identify any appearance-related rituals you want to stop or reduce, work on how you will go about this. Remember to use your SMART goals.

Being assertive

Part of having a positive body image is not being pulled down by others' negativity and particularly negative comments. One way not to be taken in by negativity is through being assertive, especially in the face of body criticism or body teasing. This assertiveness can be in situations where we are directly targeted but also where we see and hear others being teased or made fun of in relation to their appearance.

From time to time we all can look back on a situation and think I should have been more assertive in that situation or ask ourselves why wasn't I assertive in that situation? It's important first of all to know what assertiveness actually is. Many people misinterpret being aggressive for being assertive. Assertive people are not aggressive. They put their views, opinions, and needs forward in a way that makes it clear what these are in an open and honest manner. Assertive people are in tune with their needs and the needs of others. Assertiveness helps us reduce conflict and reduce anxiety and depression as we make our needs known rather than being passive and keeping them to ourselves due to fear. Being assertive can help build our self-esteem because we're putting our needs forward rather than holding back.

It can be hard at times to be assertive. For example, when we're faced with bullies we can feel silenced by them and fear putting our needs and wants forward for fear of a negative response. It can be particularly difficult to be assertive with regards to body image and our appearance issues. For example, when someone says something negative about our body or someone else's, we can often let fear stop us being assertive. However, if we don't respond to what someone says, we passively allow that comment to be seen as acceptable and okay. We can also feel bad about the comment someone made, thinking about the comment over and over and what we should have or could have said. By being passive and non-assertive in this situation we are letting the comment have enormous power over us.

Being assertive and saying something can help others understand us better and can make us feel more in control of our lives. We all have a voice and that voice needs to be heard, not in a loud aggressive way but in a way that clearly communicates how we feel about something. When we're assertive we're much more likely to get our needs and wants heard and met.

Being assertive doesn't mean shouting, swearing or being cruel back, as then it is the volume and aggressiveness people hear, not the message behind it. Being assertive is about calmly stating you don't agree and how you really and honestly think and feel.

Everyone is responsible for their own behaviour and, if the other person chooses to not hear you or not value your opinion, you've still put it forward and the other is choosing to be aggressive and dismissive in response.

Let's take the example of when someone tells us they think we're fat or ugly. They may not say this exactly — it might be a so-called innocent comment from an aunty about how much we've grown outwards since she last saw us. The intention may not have been to hurt us but certainly if we're sensitive to appearance criticism this sort of comment can be quite significant, much more so than the person intended. There are several ways we can respond: we can ignore the comment (which doesn't let the person know how the comment affects us at all); or we can smile (passively letting the person know the comment is acceptable); or we can be assertive, letting the person know openly and honestly but calmly how that comment affects us. For example, one way to respond is to say that the comment doesn't make us feel very good, which gives the person the opportunity to apologise or re-frame. Sometimes people can then become defensive in response but again we can express our needs, stating again how the comment affects us and perhaps what we'd prefer they said instead (if anything at all). Giving the other person a solution to the problem helps resolve the issue.

Here are a few tips to being assertive when people make appearance comments that hurt our feelings. Sometimes it's good to practice a few times before you're in the situation:

Firstly, *identify the problem* (is it a comment, approach, behaviour?), your feelings (be specific, how does the comment affect you?) and your approach (what are you going to say?). You might like to write it down or practice beforehand. Remember to *stay calm*.

For those serial offenders of negative comments, it can be better to initiate conversation with the person before they have the opportunity to say something negative again; stating what you want to talk about and how it makes you feel.

Get *specific* about the problem. Calmly and confidently tell the other person the particular remarks or behaviours you find negative. Stay focused on the facts of the situation and be specific. For example, you might say, 'This morning you said I looked like I'd put on weight. I want to talk to you about your comments and how it makes me feel.' Stick to a particular incident, try and stay calm and focus on how you feel. You don't need to apologise for feeling this way, it is up to the other to apologise.

The *focus* is on *how you feel* when the person behaves that way. For example, 'When you say things about my weight it makes me feel bad'.

You don't need to apologise for bringing the behaviour up; you can say you thought it was important you said something about the way the comment made you feel so you could stop it happening again. If you focus on the way you feel, the person is less likely to get defensive.

Then tell the person what you want them to do or how to behave. For example, 'I'd like you to stop pointing out my weight'. This gives the person a *solution to the problem*. Ask them to agree to this. Sometimes putting a positive spin on it can help, such as 'If you stopped pointing out my weight I'd feel a lot more comfortable when I see you'. If it's someone you might have avoided because of the comments they make, then saying, 'If you stop [the comments] then I'd be more likely to come and talk to you'. This states the benefit to the other of cooperating with your request.

As with any behaviour we're trying to increase or encourage, reward the positive change and behaviour. Stating something like, 'I really like it when you …', or 'Thank you for listening', or 'Thank you for respecting me and my body', or 'It felt really good before when you said it was good to see me'.

So, to summarise, when being assertive:

- Be open and honest about the way you feel.
- Speak in feeling and thinking terms.
- Be specific about the behaviour you don't like and how you'd like it to change.
- Speak calmly and succinctly.
- Reward yourself for being assertive especially when it may be challenging to do so.

If being assertive doesn't come naturally, practice. Think of some situations from your past and how you could respond more assertively.

ACTIVITY

As yourself: 'Where do I need to be more assertive and how can I practice?' Remember, the more you practice, the easier it becomes.

How to help your child be more assertive

We can teach our children to stand up for themselves in the same way we do it as adults but here are a few more tips for helping children stand up to bullies and those who tease them about their appearance.

Firstly, be available — such as having one-to-one time — and be open with your child so they are more likely to tell you if they're being bullied. If they start to tell you about it, just listen and empathise before coming up with solutions. The main thing is to ensure your child knows that it's the bully, not them, that has the problem. Children who bully others often do it to show off, make themselves feel better or because they themselves are being bullied. The important thing for your child is to reduce their chance of being a victim to bullying and this involves them staying in a crowd where the bully can't get to them again. Often bullies act when the child is alone. Also, get your child to come up with some clever comebacks that put the bully in their place. These are assertive responses that your child can say to the bully to reduce the impact of the bully's comment on them. Bullies often stop because they don't get the reaction they expect or the victim comes back with an assertive response. Unfortunately bullies often prey on more vulnerable children so, if your child can demonstrate that they won't put up with it, the bully is more likely to leave them alone later. The comebacks your child can say don't have to be rude or nasty, just something that indicates that the bully's comment hasn't had the negative impact intended. Such comebacks to fat teasing or appearance teasing often put the bully in their place and they will cease. For example, Bully: 'You're fat'; Child: 'Thanks for pointing out the obvious — it's genetic, what's your excuse? Is that all you've got?'

So, to summarise, when helping your child deal with bullies and appearance teasing:

- Listen and empathise, then state that you can help them solve the situation.

- Teach your child to stay protected by others such as the teacher or their friends and not be alone where the bully can get to them.
- Develop some comebacks.
- Practice with your child so they become automatic.

Many schools have antibully processes and procedures so talk to your school about these if needed.

Dealing with feared situations

Sometimes our perception of our appearance can hold us back from situations and experiences where we feel our appearance will be on show. Typical feared situations include going to the pool or beach where you'll be in swimmers, going to a party where people will be looking at your body, dating, or sexual activity.

As we've talked about previously, the best way to eliminate fear is to face it and the more we practice facing our fears the less fear we will feel.

Firstly, identify the situations in which or are likely to feel anxious. Then, identify how you would like to feel in those situations.

Often when we're frightened or anxious about a situation, we're thinking irrationally about it, thinking it will be worse than it actually will be. Remember the cognitive errors we talked about in Chapter 7? Identify which ones you're doing and then how you can think more rationally and realistically about the feared situation.

Ask yourself, 'What am I frightened of and how likely is that to happen? What's the evidence that this will happen?' Most of the time, with irrational fears, they're not based on fact and are not very likely. So challenge yourself to think more realistically about the situation. What is likely to happen? This should help you worry less about the situation. Remember, fear is our body and mind's reaction to perceived (not realistic) threat.

Write down what the reality of the situation is. For example, let's say you're worried about going to the beach because you'll have to put your swimmers on and you're worried that other people might look at you and think you look unattractive. Ask yourself what is the evidence for this thought? Has anything happened before? What's most likely to happen in this situation? More often than not, nobody looks at us, and most people are thinking about themselves rather than what they think we look like. Isn't it reasonable that if everyone was as worried about their appearance as you then nobody would be paying attention to anyone?

When we're fearful of situations we've never been in before, what we can do is use our calming and relaxation techniques to try and relax in the situation. As well, it's a great opportunity to test out the worry. For example, if you're really worried everyone will be looking at you in your swimmers, then test it, go down and count how many people are looking at you.

Often when we think about testing out our fears they sound a bit ridiculous. Use this feeling of ridiculousness to reduce your worry. Thinking it's a ridiculous worry is thinking more realistically and this will automatically help to reduce your anxiety.

Remember that we need to face our fears in order to reduce them. If we simply avoid anxiety-provoking situations, the fear often grows and we never get to demonstrate to ourselves that we can overcome our anxiety.

Sexual activity and fear

I was afraid of being naked in the bedroom even with my partner. I didn't want him to see my flabby and bumpy bits. So I'd always have sex with the lights off and I had to be wearing something. It was silly because I knew my partner could feel my bits so he knew they were there. He also gave me lots of compliments so I had no reason to worry about what he'd think. But it was my own negative self-talk and my own fear of being naked. It took a while but I made a goal to be comfortable naked. I was sick of trying to hide and it felt ridiculous when I

looked at the reality of the situation. I started off small, gradu-
ally removing items of clothing and trying dim lights at first and
moving towards having the lights completely on. My partner
was really encouraging. Achieving each step was a reward in
itself. It took a few months but I feel comfortable now.

Hannah, 36

It's not uncommon for people to have fears around nakedness but these fears can lead to people feeling uncomfortable with their partners or new partners when it comes to sexual activity. This ultimately stops them from enjoying sex which can lead to other problems including avoidance of sex, sexual dysfunction and sexual aversion disorders. When we're naked we're at our most vulnerable so it's no wonder we feel more self-conscious, particularly in new sexual encounters and with new partners. So, for some, their body image goal may be around feeling more comfortable when naked or when engaging in sexual activity. Just like any other anxiety, we need to learn ways to help us relax as well as challenging our thinking and replacing it with more helpful thoughts. If you think this applies to you, write down how you would like to feel and behave when engaging in sexual activity. Then, how would you go about achieving this? What do you need to do? What do you need to tell yourself?

It's good to talk to your partner about the way you feel so they understand and can help. They too might feel very similar about their own body. Remember that your partner may have worries about their own body even though you think they look terrific. Beauty is in the eye of the beholder so we should remember to practice with others what we're practicing on ourselves in terms of giving compliments and positive feedback.

During sexual activity is a perfect opportunity to role-model positive body image. Telling your partner how great they make you feel, what you enjoy doing, and how great it feels being with their body.

This is also a great opportunity to practice accepting compliments. As your partner tells you about how fabulous you make them feel and how much they love your body, take this onboard, collect the evidence that supports the positive body image you're trying to achieve.

> *I love it when my partner tells me they love my chest. I work hard at the gym and people often give me compliments on my muscles, particularly my pecks, but for some reason I've always felt self-conscious. I think it stems back to school when I was picked on for being weedy. I sometimes worry about having love handles but my partner tells me all the time how much they love my body. I think, 'They see me at my most vulnerable and they love my body, that's great evidence for me'. I'm learning every day to love my body even more, just the way my partner loves it.*
>
> *Mark, 30*

Hierarchy of fears

When we're working on facing our fears, sometimes it can help to draw up what's called a hierarchy of fears. This hierarchy of fears starts from fears that are lower in anxiety to highest in anxiety. Working on fears lower down on our hierarchy first before the harder ones helps us practice our relaxation techniques and makes us more successful. Sometimes if we jump in too soon and try a top fear we can become overwhelmed and not able to use our coping skills.

So write down here your hierarchy, starting from situations of low fear to top fear. Start at the low-feared situations and work out what you're going to do to try and reduce your fear in this situation. Practice it, and then as you achieve each step work towards harder more challenging steps. See Appendix B for a worksheet on developing your fear hierarchy.

Here's an example from one of my clients who had a fear of being seen in public with her swimmers on. Her hierarchy started with something easy she could achieve but was still anxiety-provoking.

For example:

1 Wear swimmers in front of family with a sarong over the top and walk around the house (anxiety rating 4 out of 10).

2 Wear swimmers in front of best friend with a sarong over the top and walk around the house.

3 Take sarong off in front of family.

She worked all the way up to her top fear of going to the public swimming pool and wore her swimmers without a sarong over the top (anxiety/fear rating 9 out of 10). At each step she'd reward herself for her achievement. She'd use her coping statements to tell her to relax as well as breathing techniques and positive reinforcement for encouragement.

ACTIVITY

Now you try. Write down a few feared situations and a few steps to work up to practice facing your fears. Make sure your steps are measurable and you reward your success. Plan out what coping strategies you're going to use for your steps too. Use Appendix B as a guide to this chapter's activities.

Make sure you reward yourself for each step achieved and remember again to make each step a SMART goal.

CHAPTER SUMMARY

▪ Reducing or eliminating rituals reduces anxiety in the long term.

▪ Plan out what relaxation and anxiety-reduction technique you're going to use as you work on reducing your compulsions.

▪ Being assertive reduces body image distress.

▪ A negative body image can stop us enjoying sexual activity.

▪ Reducing fears involves starting with smaller steps and fears, being successful in mastering these, and then progressing to more fearful steps.

▪ Always reward your success.

Chapter 9

Eating disorders

After I lost my job I started eating for comfort and punishment. At first it made me feel better, having the foods I'd not eaten in a while. I didn't worry about it at first but when I stopped exercising I started to worry about the weight I was gaining. I felt depressed and so I ate more. I'd eat all day, right up until I went to bed. After a few months I realised I'd been eating what I called 'junk' for months solid, not exercising and I'd gotten to the point where I felt disgusting. I was morbidly obese, I'd cut out my exercise (I used to go to the gym almost every day), I felt depressed and I still hadn't gotten a job. It was when my daughter said to me 'Daddy, you don't play with us anymore' that I knew I had to make a change. I'd replaced my life with food and I was obsessed with it.

Robert, 40.

This chapter covers the more clinical/pathological side of body image disturbance — that of the eating disorders. These are clinical conditions where weight and shape become the primary, if not the only, focus of a person's life to the point where the person becomes very unwell psychologically and physically. Eating disorders are marked by significant distress over one's size and shape and the way the body is experienced. This chapter will go through the characteristics of each disorder, warning signs for parents and carers, and discussion of treatment and where to go for additional help.

When we think of eating disorders and what someone with an eating disorder looks like, most people conjure up in their heads a picture of an emaciated young girl. The reality is far from this, with many people suffering from eating disorders appearing to be in a healthy weight range. There are also many who suffer bulimia or binge eating disorder who may appear overweight. It is important to note that whilst being significantly underweight comes with physical health implications, so too do disorders where the person's weight is considered 'healthy'. It is the behaviours the person engages in and the way they think about themselves, not to mention their inner distress, that make it an 'eating disorder' not just their weight status.

> Hi, my name is Samantha and I've had an eating disorder since I was in my twenties. It started with a desire to lose weight that went out of control as the goal-post just kept shifting and I wanted to lose more and more weight. It started with a competition with my flatmate as to who could lose weight the fastest. I started to believe after a while that I was only successful if I lost more weight. You could say my appearance assumption was that thin people have it all. Well, I lost it all as a consequence. I lost my job, my friends and my family as I became obsessed with losing weight. I was miserable.
>
> It was hard work, but I'm now in my thirties after working on myself and my view of my body to be more positive. Through challenging the way I viewed my body and myself, I began to acknowledge myself as a person in a way distinct from my appearance. I became more social and now am back with good friends and family.

There are treatments available for people with eating disorders and it is important to seek this treatment early. Eating disorders are characterised by severe disturbances in the way a person evaluates their appearance and self-focusing on weight and size as a value of themselves as a person. This disturbance in the value placed on weight and shape leads to engagement in behaviours to try and lose weight which often lead to dangerous physical and mental health outcomes. The most well-known eating disorder is Anorexia Nervosa but the most common eating disorder is actually Eating Disorder Not Otherwise Specified. It is important to seek help early as it is much easier to treat an eating disorder in its early stages than when it is full-blown. Often, if left to a later stage, it is hard to think rationally and stop behaviours that have become habits and taken over day-to-day life.

We often think eating disorders only affect females but that's not the case. Certainly eating disorders are more common in females but they do exist in males, in about 1 in 10 of them. The main reason for this seems to be the difference in the way the male and female so-called 'ideal' bodies are portrayed. For women it is one of thinness, whereas for men it is a much larger, muscular physique. It is important to note that this 'ideal' is a perception; in reality this thin 'ideal' is far from ideal in that it can cause significant health issues attempting to pursue it. It's not just the difference in the ideal size in how the male and female bodies are portrayed but also what is required in order to obtain these ideals. For females, the ideal figure is obtained through a restricted diet. For males, though, more emphasis is placed on fitness, strength and muscle. However, recently the male figure portrayed as the ideal through the media has become increasingly more toned and conditioned, making this figure unattainable for most men without a high protein, restricted fat diet with daily extreme exercise and muscle building. Thus there have been reports of an increase in eating disordered behaviour in men as a consequence.

Dieting is the highest risk factor for development of an eating disorder in both men and women. I work with both men and women in my practice and, consistent with the research, most people with an eating disorder can trace it back to beginning to diet, losing weight and feeling successful as a result. They then continued this extreme dieting, becoming obsessed with thoughts about food and weight and went from an initial feeling of accomplishment for their weight loss to feeling depressed and anxious about their bodies and around food and exercise. For the men, they often exercise for hours at the gym and feel depressed when not engaging in this exercise. Both men and women become self-conscious about their bodies and start withdrawing from social activities. It is also estimated that men, whilst not meeting the criteria for an eating disorder, do engage in eating disordered behaviours from time to time; for example, skipping meals, exercising only for weight loss, using weight-loss products etc.

I work with both men and women with eating disorders from primary-school-age to older ages. We often think of eating disorders only affecting adolescent girls and young women, but incidents of children aged seven have been reported as well as women in their 70s. Unfortunately, for those who have had an eating disorder for many years, the major health consequences start to show and this can be devastating for middle aged and older women. In younger females, the risk of osteoporosis is high but it is lack of energy, difficulty sleeping, constantly feeling cold and hair loss that are most noticeable.

For parents, as soon as you notice your child has a concern with their weight and size that is interfering with their happiness and the things they do, seek help. First point of call is your GP for a referral to specialised eating disorder clinics and specialists if needed.

As we discussed in the beginning chapters, it is almost 'normal' for men and women in our society to feel unhappy about their bodies and to be dieting or worrying about food and exercise. Only one in five women are satisfied with their body weight and nearly half of all normal-weight women overestimate their size and shape. Men do the opposite, often underestimating their size, perceiving that their muscles are smaller than they actually are, and it's common for them to not be happy with their mid and upper torso. It is common also for men to be watching what they eat and exercising for body shape. In extreme cases, though, these desires for body change lead some people to develop eating disorders where their appearance becomes their number one priority, often at the expense of their health and happiness.

Eating disorders describe a range of problems associated with eating, food and body image. Although eating disorders are not common in the general population, it is quite common for women to have some of these behaviours from time to time. For example, it is quite common for a woman to restrict her eating because she feels fat or because she overate the day before. It is also common for everyone to overeat sometimes. To use laxatives and diet pills to try and control one's weight are a lot more common than people think.

Diagnosis

Let's now turn and look at the individual eating disorders according to the *Diagnostic and Statistical Manual of Mental Disorders IV-TR* (American Psychiatric Association, 2000). This diagnostic tool is used by psychologists to diagnose eating disorders. Diagnosis helps psychologists to identify the condition so they know what the appropriate treatment is to take. As well, it helps health professionals communicate with each other in a simple way. Diagnosis can often help sufferers put a name to their experience and therefore better understand themselves and their symptoms. When we understand what's happening to us, we're better able to make change.

All of the eating disorders are characterised by an obsession with weight and shape. So, whilst you may know people who are underweight, that is only one of the criteria for one of the disorders.

Anorexia Nervosa

Perhaps the most well know and publicised through the media of all the eating disorders is Anorexia Nervosa, characterised by severely restricted eating, loss of weight (to an unhealthy level) and a fear of putting on weight. The body is deprived of the essential nutrients and energy it needs to function effectively, it is then forced to slow down all of its processes in order to conserve energy which results in serious medical consequences and sometimes death. The restricted eating is the most commonly seen form of anorexia but a person can have Anorexia Nervosa and binge and purge in between episodes of Anorexia Nervosa also.

The DSM-IV-TR criteria are:

- body weight less than 85% of that expected for a person's age and height
- fears of gaining weight or becoming overweight despite being underweight
- self-evaluation dominated by weight
- absence of three menstrual periods in a row.

The DSM-IV-TR criteria stipulate that the weight is 15% below what is considered healthy for a person of a particular age and height and is due to concerns over weight and becoming fat rather than a health condition causing weight loss. It is not simply that someone who is underweight has anorexia; they must meet all of the criteria for a diagnosis. Criteria four is obviously only relevant to girls who have hit puberty and have experienced their periods. Anorexia can present in pre-puberty where girls are avoiding puberty through weight loss and therefore have never experienced menstruation. This criterion also does not apply to women post-menopause, and does not apply to males.

Bulimia Nervosa

Bulimia Nervosa is the second most commonly known eating disorder, which is marked by periods of bingeing on high-kilojoule foods (often in secret), followed by attempts to compensate by over-exercising, vomiting or periods of strict dieting. The bingeing is accompanied by feelings of shame and being 'out of control'. Bingeing involves eating a quantity of food much larger than you would expect for someone in the same situation under the same circumstances. Clients have described to me that they often can't even taste the food but feel highly anxious about putting as much in their body as they can until they feel very uncomfortable. They then feel highly anxious and distressed and seek to get rid of it. They are very worried about the calories they have consumed and subsequent weight gain. They then engage in what are called compensatory behaviours or behaviours aimed at 'compensating for this eating' such as vomiting, excessive exercise, restricting intake, using laxatives or other pills to get rid of waste.

The DSM-IV-TR criteria are:

- binge eating and feeling out of control with this eating at least twice per week for a three-month period
- engaging in behaviours to try and prevent weight gain (called compensatory behaviours)
- both binge eating and compensatory behaviours occur on average twice per week for at least three months
- as with all eating disorders, one's sense of self is significantly influenced if not solely influenced by body shape and size.

Vomiting after binge eating is the most common, followed by restricting intake the next day or days later. Not all people with Bulimia Nervosa vomit after a binge, though some use excessive exercise or over-the-counter products to try and get rid of the food or stop weight gain. Often these products are very dangerous to a person's health; for example, diet pills often speed up heart rate, potentially leading to heart failure, not to mention anxiety. Laxative abuse is quite common with the dangers being around dehydration and kidney trouble.

It is often dentists who notice the first signs of bulimia. The stomach acids from repeated vomiting erode teeth enamel and cause cavities. Ulcers in the mouth and throat from vomiting can also be picked up by dentists.

Treatment for Bulimia Nervosa

Part of the treatment for Bulimia Nervosa is preventing binge eating in the first place, to stop the need for compensatory behaviours, and recognising warning signs for binge eating such as emotions (i.e., feeling sad can trigger a binge) as well as trigger foods such as sweets and carbohydrates. Working out what your warning signs are can help prevent a binge. I often ask my clients to look back at the last few episodes and work out what triggered them and then work out a plan of prevention. This might involve avoiding certain foods or situations for a short period or finding alternatives other than food when feeling certain emotions.

Mindfulness is a particularly good approach for reducing binge eating, where you try to concentrate on what you're doing and eating and then eating more slowly to avoid that 'out of control' feeling that comes with a binge.

Although people often report initially feeling better after vomiting, later they feel lethargic and low in energy and this often lasts for a few days. This is due to the depletion of essential minerals and nutrients when you vomit. It takes the body sometimes 24 hours to restore all the water, minerals and nutrients back after vomiting. The lethargic feeling is the body's way of recovering by slowing you down. People can also burst blood vessels in their eyes and face through vomiting, leaving their face looking red and puffy. Sometimes you can also see calluses on the fingers from the force used to induce vomiting. Thinking about the negative consequences of bulimia can often help people to talk themselves out of a binge/purge.

Bulimia Nervosa is a serious eating disorder that can lead to significant medical complications but is often underplayed as usually people with bulimia are in a healthy weight range or overweight.

Eating Disorder Not Otherwise Specified (EDNOS)

There are many people in our society who experience difficulties with eating behaviours, weight issues and body image that severely affects their lives. These individuals may show several features associated with an eating disorder but do not satisfy the full criteria for an eating disorder. For example, a person may binge eat but might not purge afterwards. Or a male may be very underweight and engage in anorexic-type behaviours but can't be diagnosed with Anorexia Nervosa due to the menstruation requirement. Therefore, the criteria of Eating Disorder Not Otherwise Specified (EDNOS) are used. It is actually the most common disorder experienced out of all the eating disorders. Binge eating disorder is also considered an Eating Disorder Not Otherwise Specified.

Binge eating disorder

Although not currently considered an eating disorder in itself in the DSM-IV-TR it is considered an EDNOS. Binge eating disorder describes people who eat large amounts of food while feeling a loss of control over their eating. It is on the rise with many women engaging in this behaviour. Binge eating disorder is different to bulimia because people with the disorder usually do not attempt to vomit or get rid of the food through other means after a binge. It is not just overeating, which we all do from time to time — it is feeling a 'loss of control' over this eating. Clients describe to me eating without tasting, and eating until they can't eat anymore. It causes them great distress.

Binge eating often occurs after a period of restricted food intake or dieting, so it's important to know that dieting itself can be a trigger. The foods consumed during a binge are generally high in calorie content ('junk food'), not fruits and vegetables but foods on their 'bad' list. Due to the high quantity of junk food consumed, binge eating can lead to many of the complications that are associated with obesity as it leads a person's weight to increase. These include diabetes, high blood pressure, high cholesterol levels, gall bladder disease, heart disease and certain types of cancer. One of the positive things of ceasing binge eating is that people's weight usually drops which makes them feel more comfortable and better about themselves as they can work towards health.

In terms of treatment, as with bulimia, it's about trying to reduce anxiety around eating by slowing it down, making it more controlled and comfortable and taking the secret out of it, and by helping people focus on what they're eating and enjoying it rather than eating to the point of feeling ill and distressed. Trying to eat in a relaxed atmosphere also works. At the end of this chapter are some tips on stopping binge eating if you or someone close to you needs some tips.

Why doesn't vomiting or use of laxatives work to reduce weight?

A few notes on the dangers of using vomiting or laxatives to reduce calories and why they don't work. It's important to note that purging is not an efficient method of reducing caloric intake. Vomiting reduces approximately 50% of the calories that were just consumed and less if it is delayed at all (even by 30 minutes). As mentioned previously, some side effects include salivary gland enlargement (noticed by swelling of the face), eroding of the dental enamel on the inner surface of the front teeth leading to tooth decay and bad breath, electrolyte imbalance and renal failure.

Laxatives and diuretics have very little effect on reducing calories as calories are absorbed quickly by the body. These products really only add water to our stools and so dehydrate the body, making it seem like we've lost weight. More concerning are the side effects such as electrolyte imbalance (which can make us feel faint and affect our major organs), dehydration, laxative dependence, colon infections and bowel tumors.

What causes an eating disorder?

There are many reasons why a person may develop an eating disorder and they are too complex to blame one thing. As we discussed in previous chapters in relation to the development of body image dissatisfaction, eating disorders can develop through environment factors as well as genetics and personality factors. I see a lot of parents worried that they gave their child an eating disorder. Whilst upbringing and role modelling play a part in establishing a positive body image, there are also things that are out of our control as parents. A family history of eating disorders is certainly a risk factor including maternal experiences of eating disorders. That is not to say, though, that your child is guaranteed to develop an eating disorder if you have suffered from one. What's important is that you are aware of this vulnerability and become a positive role model to your child to assist with their resilience building as a buffer against mental illness. As a parent you also have limited control over your child's peers. Peer teasing around body image can lead to development of eating disorders, so working with your school can help to put a stop to bullying. The most important thing is to be a positive role model, ensure your child has someone to go to for support and recognise early warning signs so you can get help if needed. Following are some early warning signs. Also, turn to Chapter 13 that has been dedicated to helping parents and carers be positive role models to their children.

The influence of celebrities

What hope have young women got when celebrities such as super models make ridiculous and dangerously irresponsible comments like this one: 'Nothing tastes as good as skinny feels'. Young girls hold celebrities up as role models. With role models like these, who needs enemies? The number of celebrities with eating disorders is astounding. There is nothing glamorous about having an eating disorder. Don't fall victim to the hype of being thin like some celebrities. If anything, use them as examples of why you should not be thin. What is most tragic are the celebrities who supposedly had it all and died of complications relating to their eating disorder.

How do you help someone with an eating disorder?

It is very hard supporting someone with an eating disorder, whether this is your partner, adolescent or adult child, or friend. It can be difficult to know what the 'right' thing to say is; whether to comment on their eating, body, size, shape or not.

The best way to assist is to be there as a listener, gentle encourager and support person. This involves listening without passing judgment when the sufferer is distressed and may want to 'talk out' what they're anxious about. You don't need to give advice, just listen. You can gently encourage the sufferer through praising their attempts at getting well and acknowledging how hard it is. This doesn't mean you have to offer more food or make comments about them looking healthier, just praise their attempts such as, 'I can see you really want to get better'. When the sufferer is distressed, you can be there to comfort them too.

It's important to have professionals who specialise in eating disorders such as a good general practitioner and psychologist, as well as a nutritionist and psychiatrist if you can. These people can offer the advice and assistance needed, coming up with the solutions to or the management of the problem. This leaves you free to just be there for support rather than having to help 'solve' the problem.

I often have people say to me that so and so just needs a good feed. A good feed here and there is not the answer. Eating disorders are about more than just food. They are psychological conditions that affect the way a person thinks and feels about their body and themselves. Re-feeding someone who has anorexia, for example, will increase their weight but re-feeding alone doesn't address the psychological issues behind the eating. It's very important that people with eating disorders are not forced into eating (unless a specialist has assisted in this) by family and friends as this often leads to further feelings of loss of control and can make their condition worse. Rather, being supportive and asking the sufferer themselves to tell you how to help is best.

How do parents help their child with an eating disorder?

The first step is to seek professional assistance. Eating disorders are difficult to treat and often require specialised professional help. Start with your general practitioner and they should be able to point you in the right direction. Also, call your Psychological Society for referrals to psychologists who specialise in eating disorders. I see many parents in my practice wanting assistance in helping their children. A treatment approach that involves the sufferer and their loved ones is the best treatment. We can then all work together as a team against the eating disorder. It's important to remember that the sufferer is not anorexic or bulimic but a person suffering from the condition — the condition doesn't define them as a person.

Get support for yourself as a carer

Caring for someone with a mental illness including eating disorders is challenging. The eating disorder is always there and doesn't seem to take a holiday or break, which makes it very tiring for not just the sufferer but the carer. Parents often tell me they feel like they're fighting the eating disorder all the time and that their child often appears to have a different personality with the eating disorder, becoming very difficult around meal times and causing a lot of conflict. I often tell parents to try and separate out what is the eating disorder and what is their child, trying to help them understand that the defiance is part of the condition. The anorexia, for example, is refusing to let their child eat.

The constant battle can be one good reason to seek inpatient treatment care when the situation becomes too difficult at home.

If you're suffering from an eating disorder

It's important you seek help from a specialist as soon as possible. It's much easier to solve problems that are seen to before they progress into bigger problems. It is especially important to seek help early as eating disorders can have long-term irreversible health consequences if left untreated. You also need someone who specialises in eating disorders as these conditions are difficult to treat.

Remember you are not alone, and don't have to battle in silence. It is a strong person who asks for help. It shows you've recognised there's a problem and want to do something about it. There is a list of places to gain help/assistance at the end of this chapter. Remember not to give up if the first person you see isn't quite the right match. Sometimes it can take a few tries with different health professionals until you find someone who's the right fit for you. Start by talking to a general practitioner you can trust and be open with — they should be able to recommend someone good for you to see.

For parents: Eating disorders in children and recognising early warning signs

Eating disorders are rare in children under the age of eight, even though many children are fussy eaters or have eating issues. However some signs and symptoms should always be investigated further, including:

- weight loss
- changes in behaviour with food
- appearing unhappy with body shape and size. Warning signs here include signs of self-consciousness about their body, refusing to eat certain foods or do activities they used to enjoy.
- an intense fear of gaining weight
- denial of being hungry

- deceptive behaviour around food — for instance, throwing out or hiding school lunches
- avoiding food
- compulsive exercising and a need to be active all the time
- eating in secret
- cutting out particular food groups, such as meat or dairy products, often terming it a desire to be healthy
- developing food rituals — such as always using the same bowl, cutting food up into tiny pieces or eating very slowly
- behavioural changes — such as social withdrawal, irritability or depression
- sleep disturbance.

Eating disorders are really about feelings and could signal that a child is having emotional, social or developmental difficulties. Often the eating disorder develops as a way for a child to feel in control about what's happening in their life. Eating disorders are more likely to affect females than males. It's common for parents to feel at fault and blame themselves for their child's eating disorder. Remember that eating disorders are complex conditions and often develop as a result of several contributing factors. I've worked with many excellent parents who have children with eating disorders. What's important is how you support your child through their treatment for their eating disorder.

Eating disorders in athletes

Hi, my name is Lisa and I'm a ballerina. I started ballet when I was four years old. I loved ballet and was very good at it. I had long arms and legs and looked graceful. But when I was about 12 I became very frightened of the changes that were happening to my body. I was hitting puberty and started to worry about my shape changing and the effect this was going to have on my ballet. As a consequence I started restricting my intake. I knew that if I didn't eat, then my hips and boobs wouldn't

*develop and I wouldn't get my period. You don't see ballerinas
with boobs and hips, I thought. I very quickly developed
Anorexia Nervosa and as a consequence I had no energy for
ballet. I couldn't lift my arms and I couldn't get through my
training. I had to stop my passion. I worked with a psychologist
who showed me pictures of famous ballerinas with boobs, hips,
curves and who I thought looked beautiful. I learnt that my
body will change and that this is part of becoming a woman and
that rather than fearing these changes I should embrace them.
With these changes came more energy, more strength, more focus
and concentration. Allowing myself to become a woman allowed
me to become an even better ballerina.*

Lisa, 20

Eating disorders are more common in sports that emphasise physical appearance such as ballet, figure skating, gymnastics and swimming. What's important to realise is that while exercise is important for good health, extremes of exercise can be very dangerous, even deadly. Exercising to excess can lead to heart failure, osteoporosis due to absence of female hormones needed for bone growth and repair, muscle wastage, malnutrition, as well as mental health problems including anxiety, depression, suicide ideation and many others. I have treated athletes in my practice that often present with very rigid ways of eating and exercising that damage their health and their sporting ability. They often present for treatment when their performance in their sport begins to suffer due to their behaviour. Fainting is common due to dehydration or lack of nutrients and over-training. Injuries and accidents are also common due to over-training. Athletes are often highly motivated and driven individuals and often excel at their sport as a consequence of this personality style and motivation. However, taken too far, instead of improving performance this drive causes them to become overly anxious and engage in behaviours that are dangerous to their health.

What should coaches do?

It's very important in terms of prevention to emphasise your athlete's performance as your concern, never their weight, size or shape. If you suspect the athlete is hurting themselves through their behaviour, it's best you help them seek professional help as soon as possible. Eating disorders including over-exercising can have long-term, sometimes irreversible, health consequences. Always be open with the athlete about your concern and options for help.

Some tips to stop binge eating

Here are a few tips that I've used with my clients that help them stop binge eating. I see many men and women in my practice with binge eating disorder and see the distress that goes along with feeling a lack of control over eating.

Ways to stop binge eating:

Eating regularly — it may be helpful to eat small meals regularly so that you are giving your body enough nutrients throughout the day and you are never starving which can trigger a binge. Eating small meals regularly helps regulate our blood sugar and anxiety and control binge urges.

Avoid skipping meals — if you can, try to avoid missing meals. Missing out on a meal may make you hungry later on in the day which may result in you bingeing.

Eating a balanced diet — this helps regulate the blood sugar levels and your mood, which will make you feel more stable and less anxious and therefore less likely to binge.

Have a distraction — having something else you can do when you feel like bingeing may be helpful. This may be going for a walk, hanging out with friends, reading or listening to music.

Think before you binge — when the urge is really strong, say to yourself, 'Do I really want to do this and face all the consequences that follow?'

Exercise — doing a little bit of exercise each day may be helpful. Feeling fit and active can help give you a reason not to binge.

Remember it is under your control — you choose what you do and don't put in your mouth. Bingeing is a sign of feeling out of control. So feel in control by doing something else instead of binge eating.

Relax — often people binge because they're anxious. Try doing something that relaxes you instead. Count to 10 or take some breaths and re-think whether you really want to binge.

Think of the consequences — bingeing often results in you feeling anxious and unattractive. Purging afterwards makes you feel awful too.

Make your goal health — rather than saying 'I will not binge', try something more helpful like 'I want to feel good, I want to feel healthy'.

Have faith in yourself — tell yourself you can do this and reward your accomplishments.

Reward your success — stopping binge eating is very challenging. So, each time you control it, reward yourself by doing something nice for your body like a bubble bath, massage, pampering, or putting some money (that you may have spent on the binge food) aside for something nice for yourself.

ACTIVITY

Write down your feared foods or food situations, going from least feared to most feared. Write down what you're going to do to try and relax about eating and then what you'll do to reward yourself for mastering the step.

Fussy eaters and food aversions

Although not about body image, food aversions or picky eating is a form of eating disorder where a person restricts what they will eat to the point where it causes them social and/or emotional problems including distress. For example, being a picky eater may limit their social experiences, not going out to certain restaurants or only eating things they've prepared themselves. Most adults who are fussy eaters are like this due to inexperience with certain types of foods, but can also be experienced due to traumatic incidents. For example, a negative experience (i.e., choking, food poisoning) with a certain food can set up a food aversion. While this can be adaptive at first (we might learn not to eat raw food due to experiencing food poisoning), it can later create anxiety such as obsessively worrying that food you've eaten may be contaminated and make you, your family and/or friends ill.

The best way to overcome food aversions is to work out a hierarchy of feared foods, starting from something very low in fear and working your way up to highly feared items. It's important to start with something low on your fear hierarchy so you can master it and therefore build confidence in yourself so you can move towards more feared foods (or situations). When trying feared foods, try to relax as much as possible. Go back to the chapter on reducing distress and try doing a few of the relaxation strategies to assist you here. Try eating in a relaxed atmosphere, with few distractions, and little pressure from others. You may find it easier to try foods with someone supportive or by yourself. You can use the help sheet in Appendix B to help you here.

The same can be applied with children trying little by little and going at their own pace. Try not to flood them with a highly feared food item or force them to eat it as this can have the effect of increasing their anxiety around the food and it may also start to generalise to other foods. Gently encourage your child to eat the food and reward their success. This will make the next step easier.

CHAPTER SUMMARY

- Eating disorders involve intense fears around weight and weight gain accompanied by behaviours aimed at changing weight. Sufferers experience much distress and dysfunction in the way they think and feel about themselves.
- Eating disorders occur in both genders and in all ages.
- The cause of an eating disorder is a complex interaction of several factors.
- It's important to seek professional help for an eating disorder.
- Reducing distress through relaxation and challenging beliefs about the body and self are keys to treatment success.
- Parents should look out for warning signs and seek help early.
- You are in control of your body and how you treat it.

Where to go for additional assistance

There's no shame in asking for help. You've made the first step in reading this book. Many people reluctantly seek help from professionals, thinking there's negative stigma attached to help seeking. In reality you've recognised there's a problem and made a decision to solve it or at least make it better. You've used a problem solving approach and that's smart. Sometimes we can battle with problems for months or even years before we seek help, and often when we finally do seek help it's great and we wonder why we didn't do it before. It may be that you're just not ready to do something about the problem but want information about how to go about solving it when you are ready. Each step is a step in the right direction and the first step, often working out where the help is, is often the hardest. Here's a list of a few places to go for help.

Where to go for help:

- Australian Psychological Society (to find a psychologist who can help)
- Mental Health Services in your capital city
- School counsellor
- Guidance counsellor
- Pharmacist
- Eating Disorder Foundations in your capital city
- Eating Disorders Services in your capital city
- British Psychological Society
- American Psychological Society
- General practitioner
- Nutritionist/dietician
- Women's Health Centre
- Paediatrician or child health centre

Appendix D has the contact details for some services in Australia and around the globe, where you can get help for eating disorders.

Chapter 10

Body image isn't just for girls.
Real men: Real bodies

*I used to spend up to four hours at the gym working out every day.
I was doing weights and cardio and I spent a huge amount of
money on protein shakes, supplements and sometimes I'd use
steroids. I'd go through periods of cutting out all fat from my diet
before an event such as a party to get as ripped as I possibly could.
It started off as something me and my mates did a few hours a
week with a bit of fad dieting here and there. But I got hooked.
When I wasn't exercising I was thinking about my next opportunity to do so and I was constantly thinking about food and checking my body in mirrors and reflective surfaces. I remember my
girlfriend dumping me because she said I was 'too high maintenance'. It wasn't until I was in my late twenties I really realised I
had a problem. I was failing at uni because I didn't have the time
to put the work in and I couldn't concentrate. The gym was my life
and I hadn't seen my mates in ages. I never went out anymore as I
couldn't eat out and I didn't want to drink because of the extra
calories. I felt stressed and worked-up all the time. The steroids were
making me agitated and restless, I couldn't sleep. I was having
sexual problems too. I felt alone and like a sissy if I was to ask for
help. But I needed it. I desperately needed help.*

Matt, 29

While Matt's experience is at the more extreme end of male
body image concerns, there are many men who will be able to
relate to Matt's worries. It's quite common for men at all ages to
worry about the appearance of their body, including its size and

shape. Men also tend to worry about losing their hair and older men worry more and more about their growing bellies, or beer gut as many describe it. Men, just like women, can succumb to the pressures to diet to lose weight and men too can fad diet and starve themselves to try and lose body fat. Older men are much more likely than younger men to worry about losing their looks and decreases in their youthfulness and muscularity. This concern over appearance can lead men to be self-conscious about their bodies, particularly when on display such as the beach, swimming and during sex. It is not uncommon for a man who is self-conscious about his body to avoid sexual encounters, for example. Skipping meals and feeling anxious when exercising, particularly if overweight, and worrying about what others may be thinking are also concerns for men.

Research to date has suggested that, just like women, men are susceptible to the same pressures of trying to fit the idealised image portrayed in the media and held by society at large. It was thought that men were not as exposed or as susceptible as women but this is simply not true. In recent years men have been subjected to the same objectification of their bodies as has been criticised in the research on women's body image. Some research has suggested that now, more than ever, men's bodies are objectified for their appearance rather than function. This can be seen in the way the male body is portrayed in the media. Once men's advertising revolved around the function of the male body, what it could do, but now it's about how it looks. Therefore men are increasingly more likely to suffer from body image disturbance and a rise in mental health issues associated with poor body image.

Why?

The pervasive influence of the media in how the male body is portrayed, including its increasing slenderness and an emphasis on appearance away from functionality, appears to be to blame.

Men's bodies seem to be sexually objectified now in a way that we've seen as a problem for women for many years. Where we once saw advertisements with men showing strength, mateship and handiness, we now see men in the media sprawled across beds half-naked, displaying their lean, well-toned torso or enhanced genitals through revealing underwear. It is such images that make the male body one to be looked at and admired rather than one that is functional. These physiques are almost impossible for most men to achieve, particularly as men age. We see men comparing their bodies to the bodies in the media and they see a complete contrast. No wonder they're becoming increasingly more dissatisfied with their bodies and themselves as a consequence.

We try to teach women about body acceptance and celebrating diversity but we need to focus more on our men now so we don't see the same incidence of eating disorders in men as we see in women. When we live in an appearance obsessed culture it is very clear that the message we're not sending is that everyone is valued as a person for who they are and what they do; rather, we're saying that your value is tied to your body size and shape. How often do we see our politicians being objectified for their bodies, distracting from what they do and their contribution as people instead of objects? One only has to look at the emphasis placed on our politicians where what they wore to the latest cabinet meeting has more emphasis than their political message.

Just as for women, there are a multitude of reasons why men develop body image concerns: teasing, peer pressure, family factors, personality factors such as perfectionism, and many others. Desire to feel and be seen as masculine is also a big factor, and for men now it's even harder to display masculinity as being apart from appearance; there is very little differentiating men and women. Where in the past men showed masculinity through their jobs, providing for their family, being the breadwinner, the Mr Fix It, women now do as much as men in most areas. So it's little surprise that men turn to their appearance for reassurance of their masculinity. But achieving muscularity and leanness is hard work and unrealistic for most men. So for many they are left feeling less than masculine, feeling that there is nothing that defines them uniquely as a man. As has been suggested for women, helping men is about celebrating body diversity and uniqueness as people in areas other than appearance.

So what can men do to feel good about their bodies and selves?

As we've talked about in previous chapters, it's about changing your attitude towards your appearance and doing things with your body that make you feel good; challenging the beliefs you have about your body and making them more balanced and in line with reality. For example, if you're an older male, be realistic about this and celebrate what you can do with your body, not what you feel you've lost or could do when you were younger. As well, learn to manage appearance teasing. Groups of men are notorious for making fun of each other's appearance. Be assertive when you feel you need to, as well as trying not to take comments personally. Listen to those around you who love and care about you and give you compliments, and take these on board. As well, exercise for health, fitness and fun to enhance positive behaviours leading to positive thinking. Go back to previous chapters now and follow some of the activities for changing the way you think and behave in order to feel good about your body and self.

We've also talked in previous chapters about erasing appearance rituals such as obsessive checking of our appearance and reducing body image related anxiety through positive self-talk and relaxing thoughts. As well, do things for your body that are positive such as eating well and exercising for health and wellbeing, and eradicating habits such as overeating and over-exercising, so that what we're doing is positive for our bodies and mental health. Getting help when we need it and not being afraid to seek help is also important. Men are very reluctant to ask for help so often suffer in silence. It's a strong, intelligent and wise man who recognises he needs help and asks for it.

So, to summarise:

- Be active for the body.
- Behave in ways that make you feel good.
- Think in balanced ways.
- Be assertive.
- Accept compliments.
- Seek help.

Muscle dysmorphia

Let's talk here about a body image disorder that is unique to men. While taking pride in your appearance is normal and healthy, when these thoughts become obsessive they have the potential to cause considerable harm. Body image disturbances, once only thought to exist in females, are now becoming more common-place in males. A problem only seen in men, called muscle dys-morphia, is a significant and distressing condition centred on a distorted male body perception. In essence, muscle dysmorphia is a condition where a man perceives his muscles and body size to be smaller than they actually are. Often these men are already hugely muscular and lean but are on a relentless pursuit to define their bodies even further, obsessively trying to become more lean, toned and muscular. This perception is accompanied by engage-ment in excessive behaviours such as exercise, weight lifting, dieting, and use of often dangerous body enhancement products to build muscle including the use of steroids. Men with this con-dition spend a large amount of time obsessed with their appear-ance, usually at the expense of their relationships with others, jobs and study, and at the same time potentially damaging their health. These men often talk about feeling unhappy with their appearance and selves. They may suffer from depression, anxiety and suicidal thinking as well as becoming addicted to weight loss and body-changing products including drugs.

What can men do if they think they have muscle dysmorphia?

The first step is realising that you may have lost perspective on what were once 'reasonable' goals of health and fitness. For some men, the goal posts keep moving and the more they try to achieve a perceived fitness or health goal the further they actually move away from health and fitness, sometimes leading to eating disorders. Many men can feel suicidal over their appearance so it is something to be taken seriously. One in 10 people with anorexia, for example, are male.

Overcoming something like muscle dysmorphia usually requires professional assistance as it involves radically changing behaviour and thinking, and it can be dangerous to a man's health to suddenly stop certain behaviours and drugs he might be taking as part of his muscle dysmorphia. Going through this book is a great start to help identify your goals and start working on how to change. It is advisable, though, to speak to your doctor and get a referral to a psychologist who can help. Men don't often ask for help but they need and deserve it as much as women do. Muscle dysmorphia is a serious condition that can lead to death due to health complications as well as suicide.

The key to overcoming muscle dysmorphia is the same as any body image disturbance: it's about changing your attitude towards your body including learning to think differently about your body and self and behaving in ways that make your body feel good.

What can women do?

Women need to take men's body image concerns seriously, just like we expect men to take our concerns seriously. Remember, it's uncommon for men to ask for help, so if women are understanding and open to listening non-judgmentally to men they're more likely to ask for help.

If you think a man you know might be suffering body image concerns, being available to him is a good way to encourage openness, perhaps providing some information to him if you can, or even leaving this book for him to read. There is no shame in asking for help. Often men go to their trainers and gym buddies for help around body image issues.

How to help boys with body image

As we've discussed already, boys are by no means immune to body image dissatisfaction. Boys, just like girls, can succumb to the pressures to look a certain way and engage in the same behaviours such as over-exercising, dieting and using products to change the way they look. Boys can become deeply unhappy with themselves just like girls can when they place a lot of importance on their appearance and perceive that their body does not match what they would like it to look like. They can often suffer in silence as they are less likely to seek help than girls. You don't hear boys talking about their body troubles or weight issues and it's often perceived as 'sissy' and 'girlie' to do so. So perhaps in some way we need to be more on the lookout for body image concerns in boys than girls. It's important that our boys know they can talk about any concerns they have including those about their bodies.

Just as we discuss in Chapter 13 on developing a healthy body image in children, for parents and carers of boys the same applies. Be a good role model, look out for warning signs, talk openly about emotions so your boys are more likely to come to you for help and focus on other things than body image as determinates of self-esteem. It's important not to tease boys or girls with regards to their appearance. What can seem as a harmless joke can be perceived as deep criticism and a fault by a person already sensitive to body image comments. As adults, if we practice being good role models with other adults and being mindful of the comments and jokes we make, we're much more likely to role-model positive behaviours to our children. As a family it's important to foster healthy self-esteem, encourage each other, focus on the positives, be open to discussions around emotions and listen. Boys and men are very practical and often like to 'solve the problem' rather than talk about their emotions. But like girls and women, males too need to be able to express themselves non-judgmentally. Being there and being open to trying to help is important.

We also know that active kids have a more positive body image, so make your family an active one, emphasising physical activity to release stress and tension and keeping the body active for fun. Just like with adults, kids that are inactive are at a much higher risk of developing health problems including obesity, and unfortunately it is often the kids who are overweight or obese who are easy targets for school bullies and appearance-related teasing. If you yourself are healthy and active, you're setting a great example to your kids and they're much more likely to follow.

CHAPTER SUMMARY

- Men experience body image concerns and can develop body image disturbances and eating disorders just like women.
- Behaving and thinking in ways that make you feel good will help with your body image.
- Muscle dysmorphia is a body image disorder experienced by men.
- Women can help men by being aware and open to talk with men about body image concerns.
- Parents need to look out for warning signs in their boys as well as their girls.
- Seek help if you need it.

Parts of this chapter have been published in *InPsych*, the Bulletin of the Australian Psychological Society Limited, August 2012©The Australian Psychological Society Limited and is available online at www.psychology.org.au/inpsych/.

Chapter 11

General health

---

*When I'm focusing on my health, I'm thinking about what I
put into my body to get through the day with the most energy.
What can I do to maximise my concentration, minimise my
stress and maximise pleasant feelings today?*

Sandra, 33

We've just talked about ill health including eating disorders,
what they are, how to prevent and treat them and where to go
for help. We've also spent time talking about how we become
psychologically healthy through our behaviour and thoughts.
Let's change tack a little and focus now on how to stay or
become healthy in your body in terms of nutrition and internal
health. This chapter will cover exercise and nutrition as well as
sleep and alcohol and other drug intake. There is also a section
for parents and carers on health in children.

What do we mean by health?

To start, you need to understand what health is so we know
what we're working towards. So what do we mean when we say
someone is healthy? The general health guidelines set out by the
World Health Organization define health as a state of internal
wellbeing where our body is functioning efficiently as well as
our body being free from disease and disablement. But health is

also about psychological and social wellbeing. Considering this definition, think about how this applies to you. What are the markers to you of your health? And, if you wanted to improve your health, what things would you need to work on to improve it in body and mind?

Think about what health for you would mean. Would it mean having more energy? Feeling less tired? Working out what the difference between current and healthy is for you is the first step. Once you've worked out where your health may be improved, you can work on the *how to* in an effective manner. For example, if you feel that healthy for you would be feeling more energetic and less tired, you might work on getting more sleep, eating foods full of energy, and exercising more to assist with sleep.

In this chapter we will go through the key markers of health, our engagement in physical activity, our weight, and our sleep. There are many markers of health but these are the key focus for this chapter. If we have these three areas in balance, then we're more likely to feel healthy and increase our ability to work, to play and to rest. Let's start by looking at goal setting around health and our engagement in physical activity.

ACTIVITY

Write down how you would know you're healthier? What would you see, feel, think, do?

Setting health goals

Take a minute or two to write down what your current health problems are. Sometimes focusing on what is currently a problem can help you work on goals and what you need to focus your attention on. Then, write down what your goals would be that go along with these problems. For example, if your problem is your cholesterol is too high, then your goal might be to lower it. Going back to our SMART goals, break this lower cholesterol goal down into the specifics. Perhaps the way to achieve this goal is to increase your exercise and lower your fat intake. How will you measure this? How will you know you've achieved the goal? Perhaps you might cut out butter on your bread or reduce the amount of red meat you're eating by two days per week. You'll know you've achieved your goal if your blood tests show lower results. How else might you know if you've achieved your goal? How will you feel, for example?

Your goals for health may be psychological, remember, so improving your health may involve reducing stress and anxiety or feeling better in your mood. For example, one goal for improving your mood might be achieved by exercising more for fun and fitness. Whatever your goals are, remember to make them SMART goals.

You might like to share these health goals with your partner or family so they can help you work on achieving these health goals. Also, sharing the goals and the how to with your doctor is a good idea to make sure your goals are reasonable and you know how to go about achieving them.

Setting exercise goals

We know that part of living a healthy life is being physically active. But how do we know how much to do and what's right for our body? It's important we know how much exercise is recommended for us as individuals. We can follow general health guidelines as to what is recommended for someone our age, gender, and with our physical capabilities, so we can tell if we're doing too little or too much. The reason for being physically active lies in the impact it has, not just on our physical health but our mental health as well. Physically active people, for example, are more likely to be able to cope with stress and depression, not to mention benefits to body image.

What is recommended for exercise?

The World Health Organization (WHO) has set out guidelines for adults and children as to the recommended amount of physical exercise needed for the prevention of chronic diseases such as heart disease, diabetes and obesity as well as mental health conditions such as depression. The term 'physical activity' is different to 'exercise'. Exercise is a sub-category of physical activity that is aimed at improving or maintaining fitness including raising our heart rate and giving us that puffing and panting response. Physical activity includes exercise as well as other activities that involve bodily movement and are done as part of playing (for example the rough and tumble play children do), working (such as standing or doing household chores), active transportation (such as walking) and recreational activities (such as outdoor sports, walking the dog, etc).

The WHO guidelines stipulate for both men and women that they should do 150 minutes per week of medium-intensity physical activity. By medium intensity they mean engagement in both direct (deliberate exercise such as walking) and indirect activities (household chores). This will prevent most chronic diseases. Alternatively, adults can engage in 75 minutes of vigorous intensity physical activity which includes getting the heart rate up for a sustained period of time (at least 10 minutes). Or we can do a combination of medium and higher intensity physical activity which is recommended for everyone. Those with medical conditions or pregnant women need to check with their doctor first. It's also recommended that not only do we do physical activities that increase our heart rate and increase our fitness but also bone strengthening activities (such as weight-bearing and vigorous activities) at least twice a week.

Assessing your exercise goals

So, what are your exercise goals? Are your goals measurable (e.g., target weight, length of time spent exercising, kilometres covered)? What sort of timeline do you have for achieving your goals? What have you based your goals on (e.g., medical advice, advice from a gym instructor, advice from a physiotherapist)? Did you set the goals yourself? We are much more likely to keep exercising if we find benefit in doing it for ourselves rather than trying to satisfy someone else. Are your goals realistic? Do your goals include a maintenance stage or do you aim to continually improve? Is there any room to be flexible with your goals? Flexibility helps us be realistic, as, if our goals are rigid, one slip and we might stop altogether.

Our motivations or reasons for exercising influence the regularity with which we exercise as well as what form of exercise we do. It's important to know your reason for exercise because this helps you modify it as needed. So ask yourself what really motivates you to exercise? Do you have an exercise goal? Is it a goal about how you want to look? Is it a goal about how healthy you want to be? Is your goal about feeling better about yourself?

If you answered that exercise is not about fitness, fun, or health, then you may be exercising for the wrong reasons. When we exercise purely for weight loss, for example, it turns exercise into an arduous task that we're likely to cease given any opportunity. So, for those needing a bit of a push to get into the exercise habit, try and find something you enjoy doing and can easily make part of your lifestyle. There is a section following about over-exercising and the dangers of compulsive exercising which are often seen in eating-disordered behaviour.

For those who might be questioning if they exercise too much, ask yourself the following questions: Why do I exercise? What happens if I miss an exercise session? How do I feel? Do I enjoy what I'm doing?

If you answered mainly on the negative — exercising purely because you feel you have to for body image reasons — you may need to re-evaluate what you're doing. When we become obsessed with anything or do something because it's a compulsion, that behaviour often leaves us feeling anxious, and anxiety doesn't lead us to feel good. We spoke in the eating disorder chapter about how excessive exercise is a form of eating-disordered behaviour where our primary motivation for exercise is around weight loss and body image and is accompanied by feelings of anxiety and guilt if we don't exercise. Exercising to the exclusion of other activities is also a sign that we're exercising to excess. Remember that exercise needs to be part of your daily life in order to be healthy but it shouldn't dominate your life in a negative way where you feel distressed by it or it affects your functioning (social, occupational, financial, relationships).

Exercise can be addictive because it releases feel-good chemicals such as endorphins but it can also be addictive in the sense that if the routine is not carried out it leads to distress and guilt. I've worked with a lot of men and women who have experienced an exercise addiction. Just like a drug addiction, it can lead people down destructive paths including injuries and negative health consequences.

What's important in exercise addiction is to recognise you have a problem and seek to solve it. One way is to start finding other helpful ways you can reduce your anxiety. Go back to the chapter on anxiety management and have another think about what you can do instead of exercising when you feel anxious. Remember, anxiety isn't pleasant but it can't hurt you and it does pass.

How do I start exercising if I don't do it regularly?

Don't wait until you feel motivated. The motivation will come after you've started.

The trick is to take it slowly, with small manageable steps building over time. Start by just increasing the amount of physical movement in your day. Think of movement as an opportunity, not an inconvenience. Be active every day in as many ways as you can. Park your car further away, take stairs instead of lifts, walk to local shops, exercise with friends, choose activities that you enjoy, not just ones you think are good for you. If you can, also enjoy some regular, vigorous exercise for extra health and fitness benefits. If you're a parent and trying to get your children to exercise, some tips are to focus on changing the whole family's activity levels, not just your child's. Try and do at least one hour of activity each day — remember this is moving your body, not necessarily having to go to the gym — and no more than two hours of TV or computer time a day for your children.

So, in summary, what are the benefits to being physically active?

A good balance between exercise and food intake is important, as this helps to maintain a healthy body weight as well as better mood and concentration. About 30 minutes of physical activity, such as walking, is recommended every day. Physical activity is any form of bodily movement performed by our large muscle groups — going for a walk, cycling and household chores. What are the benefits? The Australian Heart Foundation says the benefits of exercise for both adults and children are:

- improved long-term health
- improved mental health
- helps prevent heart disease
- feel more energetic
- helps manage weight
- have a healthier blood cholesterol level
- have lower blood pressure
- stronger bones and muscles
- feel more confident, happy, relaxed and able to sleep better.

ACTIVITY

What are your goals for physical activity and general health?

Where exercise becomes a problem — compulsive/over-exercising

> *I knew things had gotten out of hand when I was always needing to be moving. I couldn't sit still and was always thinking about my next opportunity to exercise and how to stay active throughout the day. It got to the point where I couldn't sleep and was starting to feel very anxious about my body.*

> *Megan, 22*

Compulsive exercising or over-exercising is when a person engages in strenuous physical activity to the point that is unsafe and unhealthy. It's also accompanied by feeling distracted with thoughts about exercise when not exercising. Some specific over-exercising symptoms are: increased resting heart rate (which can make you feel on edge), persistent muscle soreness, difficulty sleeping, irritability, loss of motivation, depression, decreased appetite, sudden weight loss, increased incidence of injury, and increased susceptibility to infections. If you're concerned you may be over-exercising, it's good to talk this over with your doctor or if you have a fitness instructor you feel comfortable going to.

Those who compulsively exercise often work out to attain a temporary sense of power and self-control and to reduce anxiety and distress about not exercising. Over-exercising can be a symptom of an eating disorder such as anorexia or bulimia but isn't always. People can use over-exercising to cope with their emotions and anxiety but in a way that's harmful to their health and often causing them more anxiety in the long run. So an eating disorder can partly be the cause of over-exercising but also participation in athletics or dance can also play a role, as coaches, parents, and other participants stress that being thin is necessary to succeed with the activity. Those involved in sports or dance may also receive a great deal of praise for being so 'fit and trim' which can fuel the destructive behaviour. This is the same as when losing weight is negatively reinforced to the point where the person loses control over their weight loss.

Over-exercisers typically work out beyond what is considered safe for the body and mind. They will find ways to work out even if it means cutting school, taking time off from work, getting too little sleep, or missing social events. Sufferers typically feel severe guilt when they cannot exercise, and rarely consider their work-outs fun or enjoyable. I have worked with adolescents who secretly work out in their bedrooms, feeling highly anxious if they are not continuously moving.

The risks with this disorder are both physical and emotional. All too often, a sufferer may see deterioration of their personal relation-ships or failure at work or school, often because they are so anxious they can't concentrate. Many who exercise compulsively become socially withdrawn.

The physical risks are numerous. A very real risk with this dis-order is dehydration if the sufferer is not drinking enough fluids. Over-exercise can also lead to insomnia, depression and fatigue. Additional physical side-effects include muscular and skeletal injuries, bone fractures, arthritis, or damage to cartilage and liga-ments. Females may no longer menstruate, a condition called amenorrhea, and this can lead to deterioration of bone strength as well as causing fertility issues.

ACTIVITY

Practice having a rest day from exercise: Our bodies need to recover from the physical stress we put on them through vigorous activity. This can be hard, particularly for those who exercise for stress relief or athletics training. But if we don't rest we're more susceptible to injury and we don't learn other ways to relax.

If you feel you may be over-exercising or feel compelled to exercise, go back to the chapters on challenging your thinking. Identify what you are afraid of (a thought) and look for the evidence for and against this thought and try to come up with a more balanced thought. For example, if the fear was that 'If I don't exercise every day I will get fat'. Looking at the evidence may be: 'My body needs a rest day to recover and help my body's response to the exercise it's doing'. This should help reduce the urge to compulsively exercise. Also, how can you reduce your anxiety when not exercising? What relaxation can you do? What calming thoughts can you tell yourself? Remember, by avoiding anxiety (such as that caused by a rest day), you are strengthening the fear and anxiety, making it harder and harder to relax.

Measuring our body mass and healthy weight

Another marker of health is our weight and whether it is within a healthy zone. Many factors can influence how much we weigh, including how much fat is in our body, but also how much muscle we have. For example, men generally weigh more than women as they have more muscle and muscle weighs more than fat. One way to determine whether your weight is in a healthy zone is to calculate your Body Mass Index (BMI).

Body Mass Index is the ratio of your weight in kilos divided by your height in metres squared. Among adults, a person with a BMI greater than 25 kg/m² is considered overweight and a BMI greater

Body Mass Index categories for adults

Category	Body Mass Index (Kg/m2)
Underweight	Under 20
Health Weight	20-24.9
Overweight	25-30
Obese	Above 30

A guide by the World Health Organization

than 30 kg/m² is considered obese and a person in this category is at significant risk of chronic disease such as heart disease, diabetes and other health conditions.

It's important to note that calculation of BMI is just one guide to health and needs to be taken in the context of a person's lifestyle. For example, a person may have a BMI that puts them in the over-weight category but they may lead a healthy lifestyle but have a high percentage of muscle which may make them weight more and thus fall into this category, athletes are an example here. It is also important to note that there are significant health risks of being underweight also. It is recommended therefore that adults aim for a BMI of between 20 and 24.9 in order to minimise risk of health consequences due to being under- or over-weight.

The table on the previous page shows the Body Mass Index cut-off points widely accepted for use among adults, and which relate to points where the risks of adverse health outcomes rise sharply.

Our weight and the issue of obesity

Obesity is a term used to describe a person's weight where it is above what would be considered healthy for someone given their age, height and gender and that puts a person at risk of disease and health problems as a result of their weight. It is not simply based on a person's Body Mass Index or size, but the percentage of fat in their body, often measured by their waist-to-hip ratio and skin-fold tests. For example, it is quite common for athletes to have a BMI that puts them in an overweight or obese range because muscle weighs more than fat. But that does not mean they are obese in an unhealthy sense. Rather, the amount of fat in a person's body needs to be taken into consid-eration as well as measures such as blood pressure, cholesterol levels and other indicators of ill health.

Sometimes it is obvious someone is obese from the way they look, but not always. So, as we've mentioned before, you cannot judge a person's health purely by the way they look. Someone may be a very large build, for example, but be very healthy in terms of the internal functioning of their body.

So what's the problem with obesity?

The problem with obesity or being obese is its links to illness and disability. For the government, this often costs them and taxpayers a lot of money due to the impact on health services. This is primarily why so much attention has been paid to the issue of obesity recently — the effect it has on our population in terms of ill health and disability. The rate of chronic disease related to obesity is increasing and this can be directly attributed to preventable risk factors including physical inactivity, poor or inadequate nutrition, excess weight and high blood pressure as well as economic and socio-cultural factors.

What's the impact of obesity on mental health?

Making the prevention and/or control of a chronic disease such as obesity a priority will reduce its prevalence. Obesity not only causes significant physical health problems but can also lead to mental health problems. Childhood obesity, for example, has been shown to lead to psychosocial difficulties such as being socially isolated from other children due to 'fat stigma', being discriminated against because of their size and shape, and this can lead children to develop low self-esteem. Parents' or carers' criticism of their child's appearance can affect their feelings of self-worth and body image and there are links between appearance criticism from family members and depression in children. Vicarious appearance-teasing (observing others being teased or observing parents making comments about others' weight) can also lead to body dissatisfaction in children. Mothers in particular play a crucial role in modelling eating and exercise behaviour to their children and this influences their eating and exercising practices as well as weight concerns.

Children and obesity

Both a family history of obesity and early childhood obesity have been identified as strong predictors of adult obesity risk. The finding that parental obesity, and maternal obesity in particular, increases a child's risk for developing obesity suggests that either shared genes, or environment, or likely a combination of both, may promote overeating and excessive weight gain in children. The prenatal and childhood life stages are identified as risk times for weight gain which is why intervention while children are young prevents childhood, adolescent and adult obesity. Childhood is an important target age for changes in preventable behaviours associated with obesity and ill health, as we know that unhealthy behaviours that are developed in childhood carry through into adolescence and adulthood.

In relation to children's health, the energy intake for children has risen whilst their intake of fruit and vegetables has decreased. At the same time, children's total energy and sugar intake, fast food consumption, confectionary and sugary drink consumption, and passive leisure activities have all increased. Recent Australian government statistics show that children's engagement in physical activity including active travel to school has decreased with 32% of children engaged in no activity at all. Physical activity is important for physical and mental health as well as sleep, concentration, and feelings of wellbeing. (See government recommendations for more information).

Childhood is an important life stage where important prevention of chronic diseases such as obesity can occur as well as the learning of long-term positive and negative health habits. Research has shown that interventions that target parents and carers of children can be effective in managing a child's weight, improving the quality of their diet and improving their physical activity levels, not to mention mental health benefits such as happiness and feelings of competency. As well, schools and childcare facilities can help foster healthy mind and bodies in their approaches to food and exercise. (See examples of government initiatives such as ACT Healthy Children's Initiative at www.health.act.gov.au).

Weight loss — what is considered healthy?

When we talk about health, we're referring to a positive state of the body and mind. A body free from illness and disease. The ways we obtain health are due to many things including our genetics, experience of injury and trauma as well as what we eat and how physically active we are. Health is also about body size, but even that is not simple. Someone who is considered underweight or overweight is often thought of as unhealthy. But body size alone does not determine health. It is recommended that for a healthy body our weight is within a certain range, often called Body Mass Index. But this is not so simple. Having a healthy body is about the internal workings of our organs, our blood, bones, muscles and brain.

What's the problem with being underweight?

Adults who are underweight are at risk of complications due to the lack of adequate nutrition to fuel the body including the internal organs. People who are underweight may lack requirements for iron and calcium, for example, which are responsible for keeping muscles and bones healthy. Underweight is associated with greater risk of osteoporosis and bone loss which makes people more susceptible to fractures, for example. Weight is also an important component of brain functioning. Being underweight can lead to memory difficulties and difficulties with concentration and attention. If you are concerned about your weight, it is best to discuss it with your GP.

Who needs to lose weight?

The answer to this question lies in asking how healthy you are and how you can improve your health. I see a lot of clients coming to me with a goal to lose weight. What I also ask my clients is the question: Why? What do you want to gain from losing weight? The majority say to be healthy but even this is not answering the question. What do you expect to happen with weight loss? How do you want to feel? What do you want to be able to do?

Remember that weight loss doesn't make you happier. It's what the weight loss enables you to do that makes you happier. For example, Margaret is a 55-year-old woman who wanted to be able to run after her grandchildren without getting puffed and stop feeling tired. She also wanted to be able to take an overseas trip. At the time I started seeing her, she was obese and couldn't walk very far, let alone run. She was also so large she couldn't fit into a standard airline seat. She had high cholesterol and blood pressure which made it dangerous for her to fly and she had developed diabetes which made her feel tired all of the time. For Margaret, weight loss wasn't about her appearance; it was needed for her survival and enjoyment of life.

Sophie, a student who was also obese, is 22 and wanted to lose weight to be more sociable and to enjoy more activities. When questioned, this happiness was about not feeling self-conscious socially because of her size, being able to do the same things her friends could do at university such as playing sports and dancing, as well as sitting and standing comfortably when waiting in lines and being in tutorials.

Both ladies are great examples of how they knew what they wanted to achieve from their weight loss and their goals were reasonable. Both did comment that they wanted to lose weight for their appearance but that this wasn't the driving force. Of course, weight loss will change your size and shape to some extent, particularly if you lose a lot of weight, and for some this leads to much more body confidence, but it is often what this weight loss allows you to do and how you feel about yourself that makes people happier, not that they have simply lost weight.

In contrast, I have clients who are underweight who want to lose more weight. What I have seen happen in these situations is the weight loss actually makes them unhappy or more unhappy and often more self-conscious as people comment that they're 'too thin'. When our weight drops below what's recommended as healthy, our brain and body are starved of oxygen from blood, nutrition from foods, and we often feel tired and lethargic as our bodies are working extra hard to keep us going on very little fuel. So there is a point where weight loss actually starts to make us unhealthy in body and mind.

How do I lose weight and remain healthy?

As I've mentioned previously any dramatic changes in our health should be monitored by our doctors. This involves changes in our physical activity, diet, and anything we put into our bodies. Some people may choose to work with a nutritionist or dietician. This ensures you have someone closely monitoring your progress and someone who can help you maintain the gains you make.

It is beyond the scope of this book to cover healthy weight-loss programs but my main tips are to focus on what you want to achieve for your health and how you can best achieve this. Always remember that weight loss may not be the way to achieve your health goals. You can achieve health without losing weight by being more physically active, cutting out excess fat from your diet, eating foods lower in cholesterol, cutting down your alcohol intake, eating more fruits and vegetables and staying well-hydrated through increasing your water intake.

How do I know if I've taken my weight loss or exercise too far?

When losing weight for health reasons, it's important to keep an eye on how much weight you're losing. Quick weight loss (usually more than half a kilo a week) may lead to strain on your internal organs. It's also much harder to maintain the weight loss over time. Key signs you've lost too much weight are:

- Your body feels tired.
- You feel faint.

- You don't seem to have energy.
- You can't concentrate.
- Other people make comments (either positive or negative).
- Your BMI puts you in an underweight range.
- You experience a pain in your chest or difficulty breathing.
- You experience constipation or diarrhoea.
- You have headaches.

Any negative change in the body may need investigating so you should have your doctor monitor your weight loss carefully.

So what can I eat to stay healthy?

According to nutritionists, a healthy intake (as opposed to diet) should include a good variety of nutritious foods. And by nutritious they mean foods that assist the body to move, think, process, concentrate, deal with stress and do all the things it needs to feel good. These include breads, pastas, fruits and vegetables. Eating breakfast is also an important part of being healthy. A lot of people skip breakfast but it's a great way to kick-start the metabolism as well as increase your mood in the morning and stop you feeling sluggish. Avoid salty, sugary foods that slow us down. Drink plenty of water to help flush the body of toxins as well as helping with digestion. When we're well-hydrated our body feels more energised too and helps reduce pain such as headaches. Did you know that it's often the glass of water we have with our pain medication that makes the headache go away?

Getting a good night's sleep

Getting enough sleep is crucial to feeling your best. Feeling rested not only helps your body function but it also affects your mood and thinking. It is recommended that adults get at least 7–8 hours of sleep per night to maximise concentration and attention throughout the day as well as help the brain store and retrieve information. Some people need more, some less.

Children need much more sleep than adults, about 10–12 hours, as their bodies and brains are growing at a rapid rate. Older adults often need less, about six hours as the body slows down.

It's not uncommon for adults to experience sleep difficulties, particularly during times of stress. The word insomnia is often used to describe someone who has difficulty falling asleep, staying asleep or waking early. People who suffer from continuous insomnia over many years are often more likely to experience ill health as the body is not repairing itself adequately through rest, as well as constant feelings of tiredness, difficulty concentrating and irritability.

Here is a list of suggestions for maximising your chances of a good night's sleep. It's called sleep hygiene. It's important to know why we sleep. During sleep our brain works on restoring our body's energy and refreshing it for the following day. Sleep helps with healing if we're injured or unwell. During sleep our memories are consolidated also. Our brain is refreshed and our mood is brought back to balance. Our skin, nails and hair grow while we're sleeping and our internal organs are working on repair also.

Sleep hygiene tips

Start winding down an hour before sleep time — about an hour before bed, start winding down and getting your brain ready for sleep. Put the lights down, get into your night attire, and try doing something that requires very little activity and stimulation to the brain. This may mean reading a book in low light, listening to quiet music or doing something peaceful. Often watching television, checking emails, doing work or study can have the effect of waking you up and keeping your brain active. It's best not to have a television in the bedroom if you can avoid it, as the light from the TV will keep your brain active and make it harder to relax. Light from mobile phones can also keep people awake.

Use your bed only for sleeping — this helps the brain associate the bed with sleeping and not with more active activities such as watching television or working. Our brains like to associate and link things, so if you spend time stressing whilst in bed your brain will associate the bed with stress and therefore make it difficult for you to relax and sleep.

Get up if awake for more than 20 minutes — if you're not asleep within about 20 minutes, get up and do something relaxing or boring with the lights off until you get sleepy again and then try going back to sleep. Again, you don't want your brain to associate the bed with tossing and turning, only with sleep.

Go to bed and get up at the same time each day — our body and brain like habits and a good habit to form is to get your brain and body used to when you should go to sleep. Having a routine around sleep and waking will help you fall into a natural rhythm of sleep so when it comes to 10 pm, say, your body and brain will naturally start to slow down ready for sleep. Getting up at the same time every day will also assist with this. It's all about getting into a routine to maximise your sleep quality. Often sleeping in makes us more tired the next day and also gets us out of routine, making it difficult to fall asleep the following night.

Get up if you're stressed — there's no use tossing and turning all night. This just frustrates us and leads to further insomnia. The best thing to do if something is on your mind is to write it down to get it out of your head and say to yourself that you'll see to it tomorrow. If you're worrying about doing a particular job, you're better off just getting up and doing it to put your mind at rest. Then try sleeping again.

No napping — a 20–30 minute nap during the day is okay to revitalise your body but if you go to sleep for much longer than this your brain will be expecting a full night's sleep. Also you're likely to feel very groggy when you wake up and you'll be putting your body out of sync and making it difficult to sleep that night. To revitalise the body, you just need to sit or lie quietly for 20–30 minutes.

Don't exercise a few hours before bedtime — try not to do anything physically active before bedtime as this will increase your body's temperature and keep you awake. Often after exercise it can take our bodies a few hours to reduce our metabolism, temperature and brain activity. So try and schedule exercise at least 3–4 hours before bedtime so your body has time to prepare itself for sleep.

Stop any stimulants by mid to late afternoon — in order for our brains and bodies to have the best chance of sleeping, our heart rate needs to be slow, our temperature needs to be down and we need to feel relaxed. Stimulants such as caffeine, tobacco and some medications speed up this process and can take a long time to be eliminated from the body. Try stopping all stimulants by 3 or 4 pm and see if it makes a difference to your sleep onset (being able to get to sleep more quickly). Any stimulants after this time will keep you awake.

Avoid alcohol — although alcohol is a depressant and so initially slows down the functioning of the brain and body, often making us feel sleepy, as it wears off it acts as a stimulant. The body has to work hard to metabolise alcohol and detox it from the body, thus speeding up the body's processing by the liver, kidneys, and other major organs. The body is working hard to eradicate the alcohol and, when the body is working hard, it needs to stay awake. This is why often after a few glasses of wine we have a restless night's sleep. As the alcohol wears off overnight, our body is stimulated to start detoxing and thus we will wake up. It is also important to note that if we've had a few drinks before bed we often sleep in awkward positions making our bodies stiff and sore the next day. So alcohol is better avoided to get a good night's sleep.

Another marker of health — our alcohol intake

When aiming to be healthy in body and mind we need to drink alcohol in moderation. Alcohol is a toxin and can cause damage to our internal organs, the cells in the body and brain, and affects our mental health if taken in unsafe quantities. A healthy diet can include a moderate amount of alcohol: men should drink less than four standard drinks per day and women less than two standard drinks per day, with two alcohol-free days per week. This is based on World Health Organization recommendations for safe drinking. However, these are just recommendations and you should also consider factors such as your overall health, size and ingestion of other drugs and medications that may influence what are safe levels for your body. Alcohol should not be given to children, for example.

In terms of body image, alcohol is also a depressant so can affect people's mood which adds further to body image concerns. It's also harder to be conscious of what you're eating and doing if under the influence of alcohol which can lead to overeating and subsequent bingeing and purging for some people. Alcohol also dehydrates the body leading to headaches, difficulty concentrating, feelings of tiredness and lethargy.

A question to ask yourself about alcohol intake is whether you feel in control of your intake of alcohol and whether it is adversely affecting your body after its ingestion. We know that binge drinking, for example, can lead to permanent brain cell damage and affects the major organs such as the liver, kidneys, heart and is a toxin to the body (hence the hangover feeling which is a sign of damage to the brain and the body's reaction to the toxin). Binge drinking for women is more than four standard drinks in one sitting and for men it is more than six standard drinks. If you feel you may have a problem with alcohol or other drugs, you can talk to your general practitioner or contact your local alcohol and drug service.

Tips for parents targeting general health of children

Infancy and early childhood is a period of life where significant cognitive, emotional, social and behavioural growth and changes are taking place. Many of the behaviours and thinking styles children adapt at young ages will continue through to older childhood and adolescence and even into adulthood. Parents play a crucial role in shaping children's behaviour including their health behaviour. For example, parents reinforce and model behaviours that children copy. If a parent is engaging in healthy or unhealthy behaviours as the case may be, children pick up on this and copy this into their repertoire of behaviours. When a parent

---

ACTIVITY

Why fuel your body with healthy foods? Because of how good they make your brain and body feel. Notice how different foods have an effect on your energy levels as well as your mood. Chocolate, for example, might initially make you feel more energised and lift your mood because of its sugar and fat content, but then makes you 'crash' with less energy after about half an hour. You might like to try charting your food intake and rate your mood and energy out of 10. See which foods lead to 10 out of 10 and eat more of them.

---

reinforces a child's behaviour through praise or reward, this behaviour tends to increase in frequency. Parents shape a child's health behaviours through modelling behaviours and reinforcing the child's engagement in these behaviours. So be a good role model and do the healthy things you want your child to do.

Mental health

There's much research to support the need for us to manage our stress in order for our body to function well and to improve our mental health including our mood. When we're stressed we're more likely to become unwell and experience negative effects

Chapter summary for Parents

▌ Eat foods for their function on and in your body rather than labelling foods as good or bad.

▌ Children learn eating behaviours from their parents, so educate them about healthy eating.

▌ Accept your own and others' body size and shape.

▌ Foster children's sense of competence and promote self-esteem.

▌ Exercise regularly and make your family an active one.

▌ Be critical of media messages and images that promote thinness.

such as tight muscles, poor sleep, concentration difficulties as well as feeling anxious and irritable. We also need to keep negative thinking to a minimum. Go back to the chapters on changing your thinking to challenge negative beliefs into more balanced and helpful thoughts. As well, erase behaviours that contribute to your feelings of anxiety and negativity. We've talked about these before but, to remind you, some things we can do to assist our mental health include:

- keeping stress levels down through relaxation and other stress reduction techniques
- getting a good night's sleep
- eating for its function on and in our body
- keep our weight to a healthy range
- keep alcohol to a minimum
- reinforce the positive things you do for your body and self
- talk to others
- exercise for mood and fun
- enjoy yourself with hobbies
- seek help if needed.

CHAPTER SUMMARY

▌ Being healthy is about how we feel and includes more than just our weight and size; it's also about our sleep, eating, exercise, energy, concentration, internal functioning and many other aspects of how our body moves, feels and behaves.

▌ Being physically active is an important part of body and psychological health.

▌ Healthy exercise should not lead to injury.

▌ Eat foods for their function in your body as well as taste and enjoyment.

▌ Be a good role model to children and make your family a healthy and active one.

▌ Being healthy means looking after our mental and physical health.

Chapter 12

Self-esteem building

Coming from a home of abuse and neglect, I didn't have a very good start to life. I spent much of my youth hating my body and myself. When I learnt that I could take my future onto a different path and have choice over my career, my relationships, my body and my happiness, I learnt to treat myself with respect — the respect I never grew up with but was able to teach myself through changing my focus. I love myself more. I was more able to look out for all the good things I do and all the positive things in my life. I have a completely different perspective and a loving relationship with my body.

Amanda, 55

Self-esteem is how we see ourselves and how we feel about ourselves. Body image and body perceptions form part of our self-esteem. How we feel about our bodies affects how we feel about ourselves. We can all improve our self-esteem to make ourselves feel better and happier. Much research has been conducted on what helps people feel more positive or 'happier'. The following is a summary of some of that research. In simple terms, the focus of feeling better needs to be on changing our behaviour and our thoughts. As discussed in previous chapters, it is the changes we make to what we do and how we think that changes how we feel.

It's a good point here to reflect on how you feel about yourself generally and why you feel this way. What influences the way you feel now and what's maintaining this? Then, just like you did in previous chapters, ask yourself what behaviours you need to change in order to feel better about yourself. And then ask, 'What am I thinking that makes me feel bad about myself? Is this realistic? What's a more balanced way of seeing myself? Am I committing cognitive errors in my thinking that are affecting how I feel about myself?'

Feeling 'happy' is a state of mind and it's unrealistic to try and feel happy all of the time. A more reasonable goal, as discussed before, might be to feel contented. Think about what makes you feel contented, relaxed or at peace. You'll probably find that when you feel your most contented is when you're doing something you enjoy or you're around people whose company you enjoy. These are often free things and things we can easily access.

There is a wealth of research on happiness and what makes people happy. There's no one thing that makes everyone happy but there are some general areas that make people feel their most content. Some of these are the following:

Be physically active — this raises endorphins or feel-good chemicals in the body. It's also a great way to distract yourself from thinking negative thoughts. Have you noticed that when you're puffed it's hard to think and stress?

Do things you enjoy — when you're enjoying activities, it's hard to focus on the negative. Even when we least feel like doing anything, if we make the effort just to get started we'll feel better. Think about the last time you really didn't feel like doing something but you forced yourself to do it. Did you feel better? The likely answer is yes.

Be in the moment — when lots of things are swirling away in our heads we often forget to just focus on the here and now and what we're doing. Focusing on the here and now brings our attention to what we're doing and away from distracting or negative thoughts. Practice focusing on what you're doing and when you catch your mind wandering try and draw yourself back to what you're doing. It's impossible not to think about lots of things at once when there is a lot going on in our lives, but the more mindful we are the more relaxed and happier we will be. For more on being in the moment you can read about mindfulness, see www.actmin-fully.com.au, also you can go back to chapter six and revise 'Quick relief techniques to manage anxiety'.

Focus on what you do well — from time to time we all get stuck on what we can't do, and what we're not doing well and often ignore what we are doing well or what is going well for us at this point in time. Focus on what you're doing well around the house, with your children, with your partner, friends, work, socially, in the garden, anything! There are many, many things we do in an average day, so focus on what we're getting done and even what we do ok at. See the glass half full instead of half empty.

Get social — there's a wealth of research on the positive effects of social support on mood. However, when we're feeling down about ourselves, particularly about our bodies, one of the things we often stop doing is going out and meeting friends. We become socially isolated, preferring to be by ourselves when we feel down. What we need to do, though, to feel better is precisely the opposite. Getting out and seeing a friend or going to that party you've been invited to will actually make you feel better. Being around others has the effect of lifting our mood. Try it and see.

Eat regular, nutritious foods — especially when we're having a bad day it's important to maintain our energy and concentration through eating regularly and eating the foods that will make us feel better, not worse. When we're having a bad day mood-wise, it can be easy to give in to cravings or start eating foods that sap our energy and make us feel sluggish. If we stick to our normal healthy eating plan, continue to exercise and do the things that make us feel good, the day will be a lot better. If we give in to cravings or get back into bad habits, we often feel worse, compounding the problem to now being a bad week and thus sabotaging our healthy living.

If you've had a bad day, though, and are temporarily derailed from your plan and goals, forgive yourself and move on, getting back into it as soon as you can. Try not to generalise and assume the worst. Just put it down to a learning experience and move forward.

Thinking differently to feel differently

As discussed in previous chapters, when we're feeling depressed we are thinking depressed too. Have a think about what thoughts go through your mind when you're feeling down. Are they negative, derogatory thoughts? As we've talked about in previous chapters, in order to feel better you need to think better. One way to think better is to become aware of our thoughts and dispute them through looking for the evidence against the thoughts and replacing them with more adaptive, helpful thoughts.

It's important to become aware of our negative thoughts because when we become conscious of them we're much more able to dispute them and replace them with more balanced or positive thoughts. Our minds are thinking all the time and often our thoughts are so quick that we don't realise they're there before we've acted on them. So try and be conscious of your thinking. When you catch yourself feeling a particular way or behaving in a certain way, ask yourself why. What am I thinking? Then ask, 'Is this a helpful thought or a hindrance?' If the thought is a hindrance, then ask yourself what the evidence is and how you can dispute it.

Write down what some of your common negative thoughts are. For example, 'I'm no good', 'I'm hopeless', 'I'm stupid', 'I'm useless' or 'I'm unlovable' are some common negative thoughts or beliefs experienced when we're depressed. Now look for the evidence for and against and try and dispute these thoughts coming up with more helpful thoughts.

Thinking errors

Remember the thinking errors we talked about before. We do this all the time, over-generalising, catastrophising, black and white thinking, etc. For example, let's take the example of a thought, 'I'm no good at my job'. If I was to look for the evidence for this I might say, 'Today I'm having difficulty with this task at work; that doesn't mean I'm not good at my job overall. I'm overgeneralising here'. A more balanced thought might be, 'I'm struggling at this one task and that's making me doubt my capacity at work, but it's one task; it doesn't make me bad overall. This more balanced thought should lead me to feeling a little better'. Be kind to yourself: 'I'm not a bad person; I'm just having a bad day'.

ACTIVITY

Write down some things that you can do when you're next feeling down. Include social, exercise, mindfulness, and positive self-statements.

Write down some of your negative thoughts and dispute them. Where's the evidence? What's a more balanced thought?

What thinking errors do I constantly fall into the trap of doing and how can I challenge these?

Things not to do: Things that deplete our self-esteem

Take drugs or alcohol — alcohol is a depressant and therefore will not make us feel more positive about ourselves and our bodies. People often like the relaxation effect, but this is short lasting, and alcohol actually works as a stimulant as it wears off, often making us feel more anxious and more negative later or the next day. Taking drugs is a way to 'escape' negative feelings and thoughts, but doesn't solve the problem. As soon as the drug has worn off, the problem is still there. Drugs are not good coping mechanisms as we don't learn anything from using them. Using drugs and alcohol as coping mechanisms can also inhibit our ability to think rationally and can lead us to make snap decisions that we wouldn't otherwise make when not under the influence. Many people, for example, report binge eating when under the influence of drugs or alcohol because their guard is down, often regretting it later. Alcohol also has a large amount of calories which can sabotage our health attempts. It's also likely that our exercise and fitness will go out the window when under the influence or suffering the side effects the next day.

It's much better for our mental state to limit our drinks to recommended doses so we keep our mind and body clear of toxins that sabotage our healthy body and mind goals.

Give in to cognitive errors — when we're feeling down for some reason, it takes real strength not to over-generalise and sabotage the progress we're making. If you're having a bad day, try not to let that ruin your whole week. Stick to your routine as much as possible and keep your goals in mind. A few bumps in the road are normal; try not to see a bad day as a failure.

A healthy mind and body: Dealing with low mood and achieving life balance

Depression and anxiety often go hand in hand with body image dissatisfaction. When we're depressed we're much more likely to have body image dissatisfaction and feel negative about our bodies. So part of learning to feel good about your body is learning how to feel good about yourself overall. There are always times in our life where we'll feel lower in mood than other times. This might be due to stress, tension, bad news as well as lack of sleep, poorer nutrition and hormones. The important thing to remember when managing your mood is trying to identify what it is that's reducing your mood and then what you can do about it. Sometimes you may just need to wait it out if it's due to hormone fluctuations in women, for example, or being sick, knowing that it will pass in a few days. Other times you may want to do some relaxation or use your coping tools such as talking to someone, doing something you enjoy and something that distracts you from your negative thoughts. If you can identify cognitive errors or negative thinking, then do the activities we've talked about in this book such as examining the evidence and seeing things more rationally. Ask someone to help you if you're struggling. Remember that a low mood is just that, and it happens to all of us sometimes for no obvious reason. If your low mood persists for more than two weeks, though, it's probably a good idea to seek professional help from your doctor in case it is a form of depression or related to a physical or mental health condition.

Self-esteem is how we see ourselves and how we feel about ourselves. Someone with high self-esteem values himself and so it's especially important when we're feeling really down on ourselves to remember how valuable we are and not let our low mood make us feel bad about ourselves overall (remember the points earlier in this chapter about generalising and catastrophising cognitive errors). Engaging in stress reduction activities are crucial as well to help us feel in control, reinforcing that we are competent people.

ACTIVITY

Ask yourself:'How can I build my self-esteem?'

When addressing stress and anxiety and working on our self-esteem, there are six key areas where we can gain self-esteem. Have a look at these now and work out where you may be falling short. See Appendix C for prompts.

We can always work on building up our self-esteem and you may like to look at where your self-esteem is lacking and how you may be able to boost some key areas.

Physical — food, water, exercise, health. These are our very basic needs and when these are not met they can cause much stress and tension. Although money itself can't buy happiness, not having money or having major financial pressures can cause stress. Addressing where you can improve your financial situation is important for wellbeing. If your health isn't very good, then this can bring your mood down and interfere with a positive self-esteem. If your health needs improving, for example, then work on this to boost your self-esteem and management of your stress.

Intellectual — this involves having cognitive stimulation, doing something that stimulates your mind. This can be anything from learning a new skill, reading, discussion of a topic such as in a book club, doing Sudoku and puzzles, something that challenges your brain. Just reading this book and going through the activities, for example, is meeting an intellectual need.

Social — this is about interacting with and being around others. Others help lift our mood, help us feel connected and provide a valuable source of stress relief. If you've withdrawn a little from friends of late, then get back in contact. Social goals can also be met through engagement in team sports, being part of a gym or club as well as going for coffee with colleagues. Having opportunities to smile and being reinforced by others are very important to our self-esteem. Our social needs can be met simply by saying hello to our neighbours or being around others such as being a part of the community at an event.

Career — this doesn't necessarily mean working; this can be study or learning a hobby. So if you're retired, for example, it might be learning something new such as a language, gardening, or something you can work towards. If you're not happy in your workplace or in your studies, ask yourself why. Is it the area? The people? The work? Whatever it is, try and re-evaluate and work out where you might need to make changes in order to boost your self-esteem and reduce your stress levels.

Emotional — lastly, for balance in our life we need relaxation, rest, happiness. We can get our emotional needs met by having contact with others, particulary around touch, communication and having people who listen and respect us in our lives. We need time out for ourselves where we're free from stress and can focus on our own needs. This is hard for busy people, especially if you're juggling family, work and relationships but it's important to put our needs first; we're no good to anyone else if we're not healthy enough to look after ourselves. Emotional needs are also met by doing things we enjoy, so finding a part of the day which is just for us is important, even if it's just 20–30 minutes.

Spiritual — this is not just religion but doing or having something meaningful to your life. This might be religion or church or meditation. It might involve the way you choose to live your life or doing something for others less fortunate. This is an important part of looking after ourselves as a whole.

So go through the six areas above and write down what you do every week or day that meets these needs. If one is missing, work out ways you can incorporate this into your life. When we pay attention to all of these areas, we're looking after ourselves as a whole and we're much more capable of looking after others. Looking after all of these needs in yourself contributes greatly to your coping in life and building your sense of importance and value as a person. Use Appendix C as a prompt.

If you feel you're time-poor or are juggling multiple things, think of an activity that ticks a few of these key areas. For example, going to the gym or doing some physical exercise might tick off a few areas meeting emotional, physical, and social areas.

So write down here what you do for each and, if there are blanks, think about what you could be doing. It doesn't have to be a big thing and, if there's one thing you do that ticks a few boxes, even better!

ACTIVITY

Work out what areas of your life are out of balance and what you need to do to get this balance. In summary, encourage relaxation and engaging in fun/social activities. Also encourage a healthy lifestyle. Continue disputing negative thoughts and finding ways to behave in ways that make you feel good.

CHAPTER SUMMARY

▌ Feeling positive about ourselves leads to feelings of happiness and contentment.
▌ Thinking errors can erode our self-esteem.
▌ Doing something physically, socially, intellectually, spiritually, culturally and career-wise boosts our self-esteem and feelings of competence.

Chapter 13

Promoting positive body image in children

I have two girls and I want them to grow up feeling good about their bodies and themselves. I don't want them to feel like I did, always thinking there was something wrong with my body and how it looked and constantly dieting and refusing to eat 'bad' foods. They are beautiful, healthy girls and I want them to stay that way. We're an active family, we eat great foods and we compliment each other. We have little screen time and I work with my girls to help them understand and be critical of media images. Sometimes I have to remind my adult friends that we don't talk about diets or make negative comments about other's bodies in my home.

Melanie, mother of two

This chapter is designed to assist parents and carers of children to enhance the opportunities for positive body image development and prevention of body dissatisfaction and related negative consequences. This may be especially helpful for teachers and others who are key adults in a child's life. Wanting to give your child the best chance of being healthy in mind and body can be achieved through positive role-modelling and proving opportunities for children to develop healthy and happy habits. There are many ways that parents can foster positive body image and strong self-esteem in their children. If you are at all concerned about your child's body image, self-esteem or eating behaviours, consult with your doctor for information and referral. Teachers and school counsellors are also great helpers.

All parents want to do the best they can for their children but sometimes we don't know how. Following are some guidelines as to how to promote positive body image in your child. Research shows that the best way to avoid body image concerns and related conditions such as depression, anxiety and eating disorders as an adult is to intervene early in our children's lives. My research and clinical work with children, adolescents and adults, as well as the research of other Australian and international body image researchers and eating disorder specialists, suggest the following for prevention and intervention relevant to body image dissatisfaction, which we will go through in this chapter:

- Positive body image role-modelling by the adults in children's lives
- Anti-bullying policies in schools and no-tolerance for body bashing
- Educating our children in schools and at home about health, nutrition, mental health and wellbeing
- Creating greater awareness in the adults in children's lives about how to recognise early warning signs of body image disturbance and knowledge about where to go for help
- Challenging media images of 'beauty' (i.e., through the presentation of more realistic body sizes, de-emphasis on negative body language and practice of 'dieting' and more on healthy eating as well as the language around fat and fatness)
- Seeking professional help when needed.

Body image issues for children and adolescents — the problem

Research shows that body image develops from a very young age, starting when children become aware of their own bodies.

Once children start to socialise with others they become acutely aware of differences between their body and others. Children are also great observers of others so they learn about their bodies from their parents, siblings and friends. They watch their parent's reactions to their own bodies and respond to comments from others, particularly once they start school. This is where teasing about appearance and weight often starts. Children are also susceptible to the same media influences as adults where they see advertising on television and the internet promoting thinness, attractiveness and other such body ideals for girls and leanness and muscularity for boys. So body dissatisfaction can start very early. Children as young as seven, for example, have been shown to have concerns with their bodies, engage in dieting behaviours and develop eating disorders. It's important to acknowledge that positive role-modelling is just as important for boys as it is for girls around body image. We're becoming increasingly more aware of the impact of body image on boys.

As a child ages they become more susceptible to body image dissatisfaction as their bodies change and they are exposed to more influences from others including peers, the media, teachers and parents. Boys often go through a short phase of relative dissatisfaction with their appearance in early adolescence, mainly because their bodies do not fit the cultural ideal portrayed in the media as they are not muscular enough. But the physical changes associated with puberty soon bring them closer to the masculine ideal — they get taller, broader in the shoulders, more muscular etc., and this can lead them to feel more positive about their bodies. However, those who remain underdeveloped or are seen as chubby or fat may develop significant concerns with their bodies and this can affect their school work, concentration, participation in sport and socialisation, all important for their healthy mental development.

For girls, however, puberty can make things worse for their body image. The normal physical changes — increase in weight and body fat, particularly on the hips and thighs — take them further from the cultural ideal of unnatural slimness. So an important part of healthy body image development for girls is education about normal body development and comparisons to 'real' women rather than those in magazines and on the internet or television. For example, parents can sit with children whilst they're viewing these images and talk about what they see, what they think and then correct misunderstanding or attribution. It is often around adolescence that girls start to become very weight conscious and may start dieting and trying to lose weight. They pick up tips on how to change their bodies through watching others such as parents, peers and teachers and have access to a wealth of information on the internet. This information is often unfiltered and unhelpful to most adolescents. Adolescence is certainly a time where parents need to be on the lookout for body image dissatisfaction as it can lead teenage girls in particular to engage in dangerous behaviours leading to conditions such as eating disorders, depression and anxiety. This is not to say that all adolescents will develop poor body image (many will be happy with their bodies), but it is a period of significant change as they start to become adults. The following tips are some ways to foster as much as possible a positive body image in your child at any age.

The best way to promote positive body image in your child is to be a good role model

> I feel good about my looks because I got the best from mum and dad; that's what they tell me. My shiny hair is from dad, the shapes of my fingers are from mum, and my blue eyes are from both of them. Mum always told me that she'd given me life and it was my choice to live it.
>
> Cassy, 12

The most influential role model in your child's life is you. Parents can encourage their children to feel good about themselves by showing them how it's done. For example, children learn eating behaviours from their parents — what you eat is what they will. Children are great observers of adult behaviour, so if you are 'dieting' or cutting out certain foods your children will wonder why and what's wrong. Try not to set up a good foods and bad foods dynamic as this worries children if they eat something that's on the wrong list. It can be more helpful to talk about food in terms of its function on and in the body such as how food fuels the body to allow us to play, study, work, sleep and relax. For example, you could talk to your child about what foods give them energy and help them think versus foods that have a short effect or make them sluggish and tired. Modelling eating behaviour around mood can also be helpful so children learn how to manage their mood in helpful ways. For example, demonstrating that when you feel down or low in mood you can do helpful things like doing some exercise, doing something fun, or talking to someone rather than eating or drinking. Children will therefore be learning healthy habits. Encourage your child to follow you and come up with their list of things to do when feeling different emotions such as being bored, anxious, sad, angry etc.

SUMMARY FOR PROMOTING POSITIVE BODY IMAGE FOR CHILDREN

▍ Talk about the function of food.

▍ Don't label foods as good and bad.

▍ Come up with ways your child can deal with emotions.

▍ Role model healthy behaviour and avoid 'dieting' and making this obvious to your children.

▍ Talk about celebrating body diversity.

Accept your own body size and shape

This is a way to teach body acceptance to children because you are a living example of how you want your child to feel and act. Rather than complaining about 'ugly' body parts or parts you don't like, talk about a part of your body you love. Focus on its function and all the great things it does for you such as your legs helping you walk, your bottom making it comfortable to sit down, etc. Also, accept other people's body sizes and shapes, not putting others down because of how they look. Not putting a lot of emphasis on physical appearance is a good way to stop body image worries. Emphasise talents, personality, values instead. If you're trying to lose weight for health reasons, don't publicise that you're dieting or that you're trying to lose weight for appearance reasons. This tells children that there's something wrong with your body and how it looks. Rather, talk to your child about being healthy, and that part of health is putting nutritious foods into your mouth and exercising for healthy mind and body.

> *I never realised that my daughter even knew I was dieting until one day she asked, 'Mummy, if you don't like your body, does that mean I can't like mine?' I threw out all the 'diet' foods immediately.*

If you do need to lose weight for your health, then emphasise this and talk to your child about what you're doing. Something like, 'Mummy has to be more careful with what she eats because she's trying to look after her heart'. You can talk about how everyone has different needs at different ages and stages and so they don't need to worry about anything now apart from having variety in their food and getting lots of physical activity so they can be happy and enjoy life. For men and fathers who might be building muscles, emphasise this as being to make you strong — again, focusing on the functioning of your body rather than it's aesthetics. The same applies if you're trying to lose weight and you're cutting out drinking: emphasise that you're working on making yourself healthy on the inside.

Be healthy yourself

Eat healthy foods and exercise regularly. Have at least one family activity per week that involves some kind of exercise; for example, bushwalking, dancing, playing backyard cricket, going for a walk or swimming. Exercise for fun, fitness and health rather than weight loss. Make it enjoyable. If you are modelling healthy behaviours your children are more likely to follow this too.

Be critical of media messages

Learn to be critical of media images and talk about them realistically. Talk about what's wrong with images that promote thinness or ill health. This same approach can be applied to anything negative that's portrayed as positive in the media, including drug use.

Encourage your child to question and challenge Western society's narrow 'beauty ideal'. Talk about the rareness of supermodels and how celebrities have make-up and airbrushing done before a photo is taken so they look seemingly 'perfect' but really aren't. Talk about people they know and things they admire about them: their personality, their talents, their kind-heartedness.

Help your child feel confident about themselves

A strong sense of identity and self-worth are crucial to your child's self-esteem. Help them discover who they are and what they can do. Praise your child's efforts rather than them doing something correctly, especially if they're learning. Always use punishment appropriately for behaviours that break family rules and never take your frustrations out on children. Positive parenting is about encouraging and nurturing children and pointing them in the right direction. Consequences for behaviour are important but punishment should never involve violence, put downs or withdrawal of love. Encourage your child to think for themselves so they feel in control through problem solving, expression of opinions and individuality. Help your child cope with anxiety and stress so again they feel in control of their emotions. For example, teach your child various coping strategies (i.e., walking away, telling an adult, relaxation, positive thinking) to help them deal with life's challenges such as bullies and school. Allow them to say 'no' to others. This encourages them to be assertive if they feel they have been mistreated by someone. This gives your child a sense of self-worth.

If your child does come to you with concerns about anything including their appearance, listen to them. Reassure them if they're going through physical changes and celebrate their movement into adolescence or adulthood. Celebrate diversity. You may like to encourage them to mix with a variety of children with all different body types and talk about the wonderfulness of their individuality.

Don't tease children's appearance

Don't tease them about their weight, body shape or looks. Even seemingly friendly nicknames can be hurtful if they focus on some aspect of the child's appearance. If you're worried about your child's weight, for example, because of their health, then encourage the whole family to be healthy rather than focusing on the child. At the same time focus on how well they're doing in other areas and give them household tasks that help them feel part of the family and contributing to it.

Talk to your school

Your child's school can be a positive environment that fosters healthy body image and self-esteem. Talk to your principal or your child's teacher about any concerns you may have. They're there to help your child be the best individual they can be. Schools should have effective practices for handling bullying, for example. There is no excuse for your child to have to put up with bullying and harassment — it's not part of normal development and it can have lasting effects. Ask your school if they have positive body image programs running and, if not, whether they would consider them.

Don't beat yourself up

Try not to beat yourself up if you feel you've been a less than ideal role model for your child so far. You can make change starting today. There are reasons why we feel the way we do about our own bodies, and focusing on improving your own body image will be seen by children and help teach them how to love their own body too.

Where to get help

If you're concerned about your child's body image and perception of themselves, then it is better to seek help as early as possible before it becomes a problem. Your child's teacher or school counsellor is a good first call. Other people who can help include your doctor, your local community health centre or a local psychologist. The Australian and British Psychological Societies have a referral line you can call to gain the contacts of psychologists in your area.

Things to remember

You are the most influential role model in your child's life, so lead by example. Children are great observes of adult behaviour. It's one of the ways they learn. So be positive about your own body and others in the way you talk and act and children will follow. We know that children are 1.5 times more likely to engage in positive and negative body behaviours if their parents and carers are modelling these behaviours.

Give your child opportunities to appreciate their body for what it can do, rather than what it looks like. Focus on the function of the body, rather than its aesthetics. For example, your bottom helps you feel comfortable when you sit down, your legs help you run around the playground at school etc.

If you are at all concerned about your child's body image, self-esteem or eating behaviours, consult with your doctor for information and referral. It's important to intervene early if you're worried; your child may be developing body image problems or is showing early signs of an eating disorder (refer back to Chapter 9 for warning signs).

Ask yourself: 'What behaviours do I need to change in order to model more appropriate positive body image to my child?', 'How will I do this?' Go back to your SMART goals and come up with the specifics of what you need to change, how you'll change, how you'll know you've changed and the rewards. You may like to do this on an individual and a family basis. What do we need to do differently as a family?

The family context — influence and role-modelling by parents

The family context is a crucial area for the development of appearance concerns including highlighting the importance or not of thinness and weight control and health. The family plays a crucial role in communicating positive or negative cultural messages regarding body size and shape and they do this through making direct negative or positive comments regarding their own or other's weight, shape and health and modelling their own body and health concerns. Maternal comments in particular have been found to have an effect on children's body image and weight related behaviours. Maternal weight-loss attempts are also related to daughter's weight-loss attempts, especially when compounded with weight criticism.

Children learn about their bodies and health through their observations of, education by and contact with family and friends. Children compare their bodies, for example, with other children their age, older children and adults. They also internalise cultural ideals of beauty from their communications with and observations of others, the media and their interactions with friends and family. Children's bodies are constantly surveyed by adults and other children. Teasing about weight and shape can start when children begin school, when children become aware of differences and 'body perfection codes' (i.e., where positive values are attributed to thinness and negative to overweight) begin. The research tells us that parents who role-model positive body image and foster positive self-esteem in their children can prevent eating and weight disturbances in children as they progress into adolescence. Teachers also play a significant role in this.

Children listen to adults talking, including appearance conversations that adults, particularly mothers, have with their friends. Listening to these conversations can for some children draw their attention toward appearance. 'Fat talk' in particular, where adults' conversation focuses on weight concerns and body shape complaints, can lead a child to equate non-thinness with bad and can contribute to body dissatisfaction and weight concerns. One way to prevent this is for adults either not to talk about it or limit its discussion for when children are not around. So be aware of who's listening to your fat talks and diet conversations. Try to stop doing this and instead model body acceptance and healthy talk.

Exposure to appearance-focused media and fostering positive self-esteem in pre-primary school aged children

There are many factors that influence a child's health including biological, familial, sociocultural, and psychological. Up until the school years, parents and families are the biggest influences on a child. When a child enters preschool, this is where peers become more influential. The family, school, and peer environment all significantly influence the eating and health habits of children at primary school level as well as exposure to media images. This is also the time when weight consciousness becomes apparent as children compare themselves to other children and teasing by peers can begin which can compound issues if family teasing has already commenced.

Sociocultural factors such as the media play a big part in shaping children's eating and health behaviour also. When studies are conducted asking adolescents about where they feel pressure to look a certain way comes from, they often say the media as well as from peers and parents. Limiting children's exposure to such influences around weight and appearance is one way to help prevent eating disorders and body image concerns. Exposure to media can lead to negative evaluations of one's body and internalisation of the thin ideal and equating this with beauty and success and fatness with the opposite. The media pressures are further strengthened by a child's family and peers and their reactions to it and reinforcement or otherwise of the messages conveyed. So limiting screen time will reduce children's exposure to media messages of thinness.

The media shapes a child's evaluation of their own body and the bodies of others through encouraging social comparisons and communicating sociocultural ideals of thinness. These messages are then strengthened or weakened by those close to the child. Therefore, as well as reducing children's exposure to these media images, discussing their understanding of them and refuting myths and misunderstandings is a great way parents and carers can help children.

To help our children be healthy in mind and body, parents and close family need to foster positive body evaluations when talking in front of children about themselves and others and discourage unhealthy weight-control behaviours as well as modelling positive body image and behaviours.

In summary

It's important for parents to listen to their children's concerns about body shape and appearance, and at the same time not teasing children about their weight, body shape or looks. Placing less value on appearance and more on health and personality promotes positive self-esteem. Lastly, make children feel that they have an important role in the family and that they make a valuable contribution.

How to influence the development of positive body image in school-aged children — suggestions for teachers and schools

In my class we talk about everybody being different and that this is what makes us unique. I don't tolerate fat bashing or appearance teasing in my class and my students know this. Sometimes I have to remind staff in the tea room and play-ground that little ears can hear them and that we're crucial role models to eager young minds.

Mary, primary school teacher

Teachers, like parents, are strong role models for children. So the same principals described above for parents are relevant to teachers. For schools, it's important to promote respect towards others. When we respect others we don't bully or make fun of others for their differences. Many schools have overarching principles of treating others well and with respect and there are penalties for breaking this rule. It's important early on that children learn that prejudice will not be tolerated and that acts of kindness towards each other are fostered instead.

We know that 25–30% of children are teased at school for their weight, in particular for being fat, even those who are a healthy weight. This teasing makes children 1.5 times more likely to binge eat or diet for weight loss, which shows the powerful influence of teasing. About half of primary school aged girls are dieting and one-third of both boys and girls in Western cultures are engaging in weight-loss behaviours due to concern over the way they look.

I've heard horror stories of children being weighed in class and the whole class finding out who is the fattest and thinnest with numbers and figures being put on the board. This behaviour can be very damaging to children as they're being publicly humiliated. When children need to be weighed, it is much better to do this in private. Even pointing out children's differing heights can lead some vulnerable children to develop body image concerns. As a parent it is reasonable to refuse to subject your child to such public activities. Of course, this not only relates to body image — differences in academic ability should also be kept private. Children can unintentionally cause each other significant distress if they make jokes about each other and point out differences in a negative manner. Yes, children will naturally do this to some extent, but as adults we have a role in modelling appropriate behaviour and minimising the chances of bullying. Celebrating body diversity is a way that schools can help children form positive body image and respect each other's bodies.

Schools are good avenues for reaching parents and so consideration may be made to educating parents in school bulletins and information nights about how they can promote positive body image and mental health in their children.

When promoting health in children it's important to de-emphasise weight and size, particularly with all the emphasis on obesity recently. A focus on children's weight and size as a marker of health is counterproductive to fostering positive body image and promoting celebration of body diversity. As much as possible, avoid behaviours that centre on children's weight, shape and size, especially where comparisons can be made. This only highlights children's attention in a negative way to the negative associations of overweight and obesity.

Preventing weight concerns among children, particularly as they commence school and become influenced by peers, is also an important area to target for ensuring resilience and good mental health as children develop. Preventative work such as resilience building and celebrating body diversity as well as the effects of teasing are important to prevent body image concerns developing into more serious mental health problems including eating disorders. In schools, programs focusing on healthy eating, body image and self-esteem building have shown positive results in the research and can be adopted by schools aiming at behaviour and attitudinal change. Schools that encourage active time during breaks have reported children being more physically active.

In schools, teaching fitness and physical activity, generally celebrating body diversity (accepting people of all shapes and sizes), and aiming physical education classes at all fitness levels so as not to isolate those children who may be overweight or less active and fit then others, is important. Focus less on competition between peers, and instead emphasise success as taking part and trying one's best. Certainly less of a focus on individual children being on public display when involved in fitness and health activities is necessary, as this can affect children's self-esteem. Challenge teacher and parent perceptions of thin equals beautiful and thin equals health. Rather, celebrate diversity in body size and shape and equate health with other measures other than looks. As well, teacher and parent training on positive role-modelling and body acceptance is useful. No bullying policies should also be adopted in schools, particularly in relation to 'fat bashing'.

> *As a high school teacher, I see a lot of peer teasing particularly around appearance. It's often about weight and sometimes height. I also see students trying to live up to ideals in the media and we have our fair share of girls with eating disorders at our school. It's sad to see such a waste of energy going towards worry about size and shape, particularly by the girls. I run a positive body image class at the school where I help the students become more critical of media messages. As well, helping students understand the dangers of eating disorders and where they can go to get help. Our school also sends information out to parents so they know what their children are being taught.*
>
> *Sally, high school teacher*

For further assistance for schools see the Australian, UK and USA Government reports on promoting health and positive body image.

In summary, whether a parent, teacher or carer of children, being a positive role model is crucial to demonstrating to children how to behave towards their own and others' bodies — treating oneself and each other with respect and dignity. Of course, if you are worried about a child, talking to someone who can help is crucial and it's important to raise the issue before it requires intervention. Prevention is the key.

Activity

Ask yourself: 'What does your school do to promote positive body image?' How can you as a teacher promote positive body image amongst your class? What do you need to be aware of in your own behaviour to ensure you're a positive role model to the children under your care?

Chapter summary

- Be a good role model in your own behaviour and attitude and promote the behaviours you want to see in your children.
- Talk positively about people's bodies, especially around children.
- Make your family an active one.
- Talk to your school and make it a safe place for children, free from appearance teasing.
- Foster positive self-esteem in your child through encouraging talents, hobbies, qualities and kindness.
- Be open to talking to your child about their worries and troubles in a non-judgmental way.
- Help your child to find solutions to their problems.
- Praise and encourage your child.
- Never use physical punishment.
- Set yourself some SMART goals and reward your and your family's success!

Chapter 14

Loving the skin you're in: Finishing up

By loving myself and my body I'm saying to the world I'm important and valuable and I deserve to be treated with respect and dignity. The change in my behaviour and attitude helps me greet each day with optimism and hope in ways that others close to me have noticed. My friends and family say that I'm fun to be around and make them feel good too.

Anna, 24

In the previous chapters you learnt not just to question your thoughts but to look at the evidence that does or does not support them. By considering our thoughts more objectively and trying to come up with balanced thoughts, we're more likely to question our negativity and accept the positive. Some of our thoughts can be easily disputed when we really think about whether there's any validity to them. Recognising when we commit cognitive errors also helps us see our lives and selves in more balance. Remember, thoughts are not facts. Thoughts are our interpretation of the world around us. Thoughts are influenced by our experiences and thoughts can be real and imagined. So, question the thoughts you have rather than blindly accepting them. When we question our beliefs, this helps us throw out those that aren't useful or are harmful and replace them with more helpful thoughts and beliefs. So next time you catch yourself feeling bad about your body or self, ask yourself,

'What thought is contributing to this?' Then, 'Is this thought valid and reliable?' If not, throw it out. If there is some validity to it, then question if there's a more balanced way to see it, a way that doesn't make you feel unnecessarily bad.

As mentioned before, changing our beliefs is hard and it can take a lot of practice to change them. We need to collect lots of evidence against them and in support of more helpful beliefs. We also need to behave in ways that support our more balanced or different beliefs. So if you believe you are ugly, you need to do and say things that go against this. What can I do that makes me feel beautiful? What can I say to myself that makes me believe I'm beautiful?

We've talked about the importance of behaving in ways that make us feel healthy and positive in our bodies and minds. These have included getting enough sleep, keeping stress levels down through relaxation, feeding our bodies so they function well, cutting down on negative behaviours such as eating for emotional reasons, and cutting down or out completely alcohol and drugs. Hopefully you've set yourself some goals around your health that you can keep working on. Making lifestyle choices that support your body and mind long-term are positive ways to keep yourself away from stress and anxiety as well as increasing your mood and wellbeing. This may involve erasing ritualistic behaviours that pull us down as well as facing anxiety and fear through positive self-talk, being assertive and taking compliments.

Treat your body like it's your best friend.

Now let's go back to looking at our behaviour. Our body is the only one we're given and we have it lifelong. So treat it right. Ask yourself, 'How do I treat my best friend?' You probably say complimentary things to him/her; spend time doing enjoyable things with them; buy them presents and gifts; and you're never horrible or say nasty things to them. So why not treat your body this way? If your body was your best friend, what would you say to it and do with it?

Treating your body like it's your best friend means you take it out, show it off, give it compliments and do nice things with it. If your body was your best friend you'd never tell it it's ugly or isn't good enough. It wouldn't be your best friend if you did.

So try this experiment — for one day treat your body like it's your best friend. Take it shopping, buy it something nice, give it compliments, make it feel good through a bath or wearing something that feels nice and then thank it for always being there for you. Ask yourself what you would say to your friend if she/he was having a bad day with their body and do this to yourself.

Ask yourself, 'If I was to treat my body well, what would I do? What would I say to it? How would I think? How would I feel?' Use the previous chapters on positive behaviours and positive thinking for the body to work out how you can treat your body and mind well.

For men

Treating your body like it's your best friend might seem a bit feminine but men need to treat their bodies well and with compliments just like women do. The things that make your body feel good might include doing some exercise, lifting weights, going for a run — something that engages your body to get the endorphins or feel-good chemicals going. Other things that make men's bodies feel good are doing other physical things such as household chores like fixing things around the home, car or garden to give you a sense of achievement.

Men just like women like pampering. So take yourself off for a massage or get your partner to give you one. Also, treatments such as pedicures and foot massages make men feel wonderful. Getting your hair cut and having a head massage at the hairdressers are great ways to relieve stress and enhance your appearance. Wearing nice-feeling fabrics or your favourite cologne will give you more body confidence because you are engaging your senses of touch and smell.

Sexual activity is another feel-good activity for our bodies where we engage ourselves in pleasure. Being swept away in the moment is great for stress release as well as improving body self-consciousness. Focusing on the here and now and what you're doing rather than how you look will enhance your pleasure. This goes for both genders.

Also, take note of the attention you may get from your partner or someone you're attracted to. And notice the looks or comments you may get from mates or strangers. Often men joke with each other, making fun of each other's appearance, but this is often a sign of admiration rather than belittlement.

Preparing for setbacks

We can't be perfect all of the time and, when we're working towards goals, sometimes we move forwards and backwards while we try to find the right balance and learn new behaviours and ways of being. It's important to realise that we all have setbacks such as not being able to exercise or eating things we'd prefer not to, or having a bad body image day. It is normal and natural to have setbacks and it's important to recognise this. What we need to do is not let a setback deter us from continuing to move forward. A slip here and there is normal. We need to learn and just move on from it. So if you've had a day where you've derailed from your plan, don't beat yourself up over it, just start again from what you had been doing before.

Many people let a slip turn into a relapse or complete collapse, derailing them from their goals. How many of us after eating something on our 'bad list' then tell ourselves we've blown it and then sabotage our efforts by continuing to eat the 'bad food', feeling guilty and bad about ourselves. Instead, say to yourself, 'I've had a slip and that's all'. This slip is a reminder that we need to stay focused on our goals and we're not perfect. But we can just start back again right now. So put the 'bad food' down and move forwards.

How many of us have derailed on our 'diet' with a little slip, and then told ourselves we've blown it so we might as well eat a whole pile of the foods we've deprived ourselves of and start again tomorrow? I say, once you've noticed the slip, why not start again now? Don't wait for tomorrow — just get back into healthy habits right now. There's no reason why it has to wait until tomorrow and you don't need to punish yourself for a slip-up.

Try not to feel guilty about your slip, although this is normal. Try and see it instead as a learning experience and get back going on what you were doing before. This will lead to more of a positive approach and you teaching yourself that when you fall you can pick yourself right back up again.

Accepting compliments

How do you think you would feel if you actually believed the compliments you've received from people over the years and thought about them regularly? Happy? Content? Complimentary of yourself? We're too often quick to dismiss positive comments from others and rather tune in to negative comments or feedback. For example, we're more likely to focus on how ugly we think we look trying on clothes than take on the positive comment our friend makes, 'That outfit really suits you'. Practice taking note of all the compliments you receive, record them, and try and focus on and believe them.

Beliefs take time to change and we often need a lot of evidence to the contrary to change our beliefs. So collect as much evidence as you can that supports your positive body parts and looks. Take note of the comments others make to you in person, on cards and letters. Try and really consider the comments and take them on board as they were intended.

Write down any compliments you can remember receiving and look out for them every day. Give others compliments also and you're more likely to receive them in return.

Stop thinking about stereotypes

People come in all shapes and sizes and there is no one perfect or ideal body; even the bodies in the media portrayed as ideal vary in size and shape. Stop comparing yourself to those in the media; no real person looks like that so we shouldn't aspire to look a way that is unrealistic and unattainable. Look around in public at people's bodies — they're all different. Learn to appreciate body diversity, yours and others. When we accept others' bodies as beautiful, it helps us accept our own. What makes your body unique?

No-one is perfect, although we might think they are

Remember, body perceptions are in our heads, not on your physical body. Through media literacy we learn that images of models and celebrities in magazines are significantly touched-up to get rid of so called 'imperfections'. So not even models have perfect bodies and these bodies portrayed in the media are certainly nowhere near 'real' bodies. The celebrity Cindy Crawford was famous for saying, 'Not even I wake up in the morning looking like Cindy Crawford', implying that a lot of effort goes into how she looked when modelling.

Rewarding your hard work

One of the most important things we can do in order to keep us motivated towards our goals is celebrating our steps towards them. Being happy with our progress is important so celebrate every step in the right direction. Often we only reward ourselves when we actually achieve the goal 100%, but this achievement can sometimes take a long time depending on the goal. For example, if your goal is to be able to run up a flight of stairs and you're just starting to walk after an injury, being able to run, let alone up a flight of stairs, might take a few months if not longer to achieve. That's a long time to wait until your reward yourself. A better way is to break the achievement up into smaller steps such as being able to do walking, then walk for a period of time, then walk up the stairs, and so on. To keep yourself motivated, celebrate every small step as a huge achievement towards your overall goal.

Rewards keep us motivated and may be intrinsic or extrinsic. Intrinsic rewards are those that come from within such as feeling good, feeling a sense of achievement or feeling proud of yourself. Extrinsic rewards are those that come from the external environment such as gifts or things we might do for ourselves. Extrinsic rewards are rewards we can see or hear, whereas intrinsic ones are the way we feel or think. Decide what sort of reward you'd like and what will motivate you the most. For some, knowing you have achieved a goal or step may be reward enough but for others you may need something tangible such as doing something nice for yourself or receiving praise from others. Our bodies and minds work hard and need to be rewarded for their efforts.

ACTIVITY

Write down what are the small steps you are taking towards your positive body image and what you'll do to reward yourself for the achievement. Remember to make your goals SMART goals and set rewards frequently so you're encouraged to keep going all the way.

Conclusion

Throughout this book you've learnt how to change the way you think, feel and behave towards your body with the aim of improving your body image. These lessons will take time to learn and you will need to continue to regularly challenge the way you think about and behave towards your body throughout your life for lasting change. At any point you can go back to the exercises you've been taught and keep working towards your goals. You may find that every now and then you want to revisit your goals and develop new ones.

If you're a parent or educator, having a positive body image yourself will make you an excellent role model for children and young people as well as your friends and family members. Stop and think before you speak and try to make more positive comments about people's talents and uniqueness. This will help you focus less on looks which will help you be a better role model to others.

For helpers, you may want to go through this with your clients, children or friends to help them have a more positive body image and live a healthier and happier life.

Keep it up and remember to love the skin you're in!

References

References on relaxation

Davis, M., Eshelman, M. & McKay, E.R. (2000). *The Relaxation and Stress Reduction Workbook*. Oakland, USA: New Harbinger Publications.

Kabat-Zinn, J. (1990). *Full Catastrophe Living*. New York, USA: DeltaPublications.

Lovell, T. (2006). *Progressive Muscle Relaxation*. Georgia, USA: Counselling and Career Development Centre, Georgia Southern University. Available online http://students.georgiasouthern.edu/counseling

Practitioner-oriented publications on body image therapy

Cash, T.F. (2003). Body image: Learning to like your looks and yourself. *Eating Disorders Today, 1 (5),* pp. 1, 12–13.

Cash, T.F. (2002). The management of body image problems. In C. Fairburn & K. Brownell (eds), *Eating Disorders and Obesity: A Comprehensive Handbook*, 2nd edn, pp. 599–603. New York: Guilford Press.

Cash, T.F. & Strachan, M.D. (2002). Cognitive behavioural approaches to changing body image. In T.F. Cash & T. Pruzinsky (eds), *Body Image: A Handbook of Theory, Research, and Clinical Practice*, pp. 478–486. NY: Guilford Press.

Cash, T.F. & Strachan, M.D. (1999). Body images, eating disorders, and beyond. In R. Lemberg (ed.), *Eating Disorders: A Reference Sourcebook*, pp. 27–36. Phoenix, AZ: Oryx Press.

Devaraj, S. & Lewis, V. (2010). Enhancing positive body image in women. An evaluation of a group intervention program. *Journal of Applied Biobehavioural Research, 15*(02), 103–116

InPsych, the Bulletin of the Australian Psychological Society Limited, August 2012©The Australian Psychological Society Limited, available online at www.psychology.org.au/inpsych/.

State of Victoria, Department of Human Services, (2002). *Research Review of Body Image Programs. An Overview of Body Image Dissatisfaction Prevention Interventions* by Susan J Paxton, Body Image and Health Inc and Psychology Department, University of Melbourne. Prepared for the Victorian Government Department of Human Services. Melbourne Victoria. http://www.health.vic.gov.au/health-promotions/downloads/research_review.pdf.

References on eating disorders

American Psychiatric Association Work Group on Eating Disorders (2000). Practice guideline for the treatment of patients with eating disorders (revision). *American Journal of Psychiatry*, 2000; 157(1 Suppl): 1–39.

American Psychiatric Association (2000). Diagnostic and Statistical Manual for Mental Disorders, fourth edition (DSM-IV-TR). Washington, DC: American Psychiatric Press.

Apple R.F. & Agras W.S. (1997). Overcoming eating disorders. A cognitive-behavioral treatment for bulimia and binge-eating disorder. San Antonio: Harcourt Brace & Company.

Butterfly Fundation. http://thebutterflyfundation.org.au.

National Centre for Eating Disorders. http://eating-disorders.org.uk.

References on body image and obesity research

McCabe, M.P., Fuller-Tyszkiewicz, M., Mellor, D., Ricciardelli, L., Skouteris, H. & Mussap, A. (2011). Body satisfaction among adolescents in eight different countries, *Journal of Health Psychology*, pp. 1–9.

McCabe, M.P., Mavoa, H., Ricciardelli, L.A., Schultz, J.T., Waqa, G. & Fotu, K.F. (2011). Socio-cultural agents and their impact on body image and body change strategies among adolescents in Fiji, Tonga, Tongans in New Zealand and Australia, *Obesity Reviews*, vol. 12, Supplement 2, pp. 61–67.

McPhie, S., Skouteris, H., McCabe, M., Ricciardelli, L., Milgrom, J., Baur, L., Aksan, N. & Dell'Aquila, D. (2011). Maternal correlates of preschool child eating behaviours and Body Mass Index: A cross-sectional study, *International Journal of Pediatric Obesity*, vol. 6, no. 5–6, pp. 476–480, Wiley, Blackwell.

Mitchell, J., Skouteris, H., McCabe, M., Ricciardelli, L.A., Milgrom, J., Baur, L.A., Fuller-Tyszkiewicz, M. & Dwyer, G. (2011). Physical activity in young children: A systematic review of parental influences, *Early Child Development and Care*, pp. 1–27, Routledge, Abingdon, England.

Skouteris, H., McCabe, M., Ricciardelli, L.A., Milgrom, J., Baur, L.A., Aksan, N. & Dell-Aquila, D. (2011). Parent–child interactions and obesity prevention: A systematic review of the literature. *Early Child Development and Care*, pp. 1–22.

Mellor, D., Fuller-Tyszkiewicz, M., McCabe, M.P. & Ricciardelli, L.A. (2010). Body image and self-esteem across age and gender: A short-term longitudinal study, *Sex Roles*, vol. 63, no. 9–10, pp. 672–681.

References on children's body image, general and mental health

ABS (Australian Bureau of Statistics) (2001). *Children's participation in cultural and leisure activities, Australia*. ABS.

Australian Bureau of Statistics (2009). National Health Survey: Summary of Results, Australian Bureau of Statistics, Australia.

Anderson, N & Wold, B. (1992). Parental and peer influences on leisure-time physical activity in young adolescents. *Research Quarterly for Exercise and Sport* 63(4):341–8.

Annus, A.M., Smith, G.T., Masters, K. (2008). Manipulation of thinness and restricting expectancies: Further evidence for a causal role of thinness and restricting expectancies in the etiology of eating disorders. *Psychology of Addictive Behaviors*, 22(2), 278–287. doi: 10.1037/0893-164X.22.2.278

Ata, R.N., Ludden, A.B. & Lally, M.M. (2007). The Effects of Gender and Family, Friends, and Media Influences on Eating Behaviors and Body Image during Adolescence. *Journal of Youth and Adolescence, 36 (8),* 1024–1037.

Baumeister, S.B. & Roy F. (ed.) (1993). Causes and consequences of low self-esteem in children and adolescents. Self-esteem: The puzzle of low self-regard. New York: Plenum Press.

Birch L.L (1999). Development of food preferences. *Annual Review of Nutrition 19*, 41–62.

Birch, L.L. & Fisher, J.O. (2000). Mothers' child-feeding practices influence daughters' eating and weight. *American Journal of Clinical Nutrition, 71*, 1054–1061.

Booth, M., Chey, T., Wake, M., Norton, K., Hesketh, K., Dollman, J. & Robertson, I. (2003). Change in the prevalence of overweight and obesity among young Australians, 1969–1997. *American Journal of Clinical Nutrition* 77:29–36.

Booth, M., Wake, M., Armstrong, T., Chey, T., Hesketh, K. & Mathur, S. (2001). The epidemiology of overweight and obesity among Australian children and adolescents, 1995–97. *Australian and New Zealand Journal of Public Health* 25(2):162–9.

Cash, T., F. & Pruzinsky, T. (2004). *Body Image: A Handbook of Theory, Research and Clinical Practice.* USA: Guildford Press.

Cherene, K., Ricciardelli, L. & Clarke, J. (1999). Problem eating attitudes and behaviours in young children. *International Journal of Eating Disorders, 25*(3), 281–286.

Cole T.J., Bellizzi, M.C., Flegal, K.M. & Dietz, W.H. (2000). Establishing a standard definition for child overweight and obesity worldwide: International survey. *British Medical Journal, 320,* 1–6.

Cook T., Coles-Rutishauser, I. & Seelig, M. (2001). *Comparable data on food and nutrient intake and physical measurements from the 1983, 1985 and 1995 national surveys.* Canberra. Commonwealth Department of Health and Ageing.

Cooke, L. (2004). The development and modification of children's eating habits. *British Nutrition Foundation Nutrition Bulletin, 29,* 31–35.

Cooley, E., Toray, T., Chuan Wang, M. & Valdez, N.N (2008). Maternal effects on daughters' eating pathology and body image. *Eating Behaviours, 9,* 52–61.

Coombs, R.H, Paulson, M, J. & Richardson, M.A. (1991). Peer vs parental influence in substance use among Hispanic and Anglo children and adolescents. *Journal of Youth and Adolescence, 20, (1),* 73–88. doi: 10.1007/BF01537352.

Cutting, T.M., Fisher, J.O., Grimm, T.K. & Birch, L.L. (1999). Like mother, like daughter: Familial patterns of overweight are mediated by mother's dietary disinhibition. *American Journal of Clinical Nutrition, 69,* 608–613.

Davison, K.K. & Birch, L.L. (2001). Child and parent characteristics as predictors of change in girls' body mass index. *International Journal of Obesity,* 25 (1) 1,834–1,842

Davis, M., Baranowski, T., Doyle, C. (1998). Environmental influences on dietary behavior among children: Availability and accessibility of fruits and vegetables enable consumption. *Journal of Health Education, 29, 26–32.*

Deal, T.B. (1993). Physical activity patterns of preschoolers during a developmental movement program. *Child Study Journal, 23* (3), 115–133.

Devaraj, S. & Lewis, V. (2010). Enhancing positive body image in women. An evaluation of a group intervention program. *Journal of Applied Biobehavioural Research, 15 (2), 103–116.*

Dohnt, H.K. & Tiggemann, M. (2006). The contribution of peer and media influences to the development of body satisfaction and self-esteem in young girls: A prospective study. *Developmental Psychology, 42*(5), 929–936.

Diaz, S.C. (2005). Coaches, parents and administrators need to foster emotional growth for youth through sports. *Child Study Journal, 23* (3), 115–133.

Dixon, J., Eckersley, R. & Banwell, C. (2003). The big picture: The economic and socio-cultural determinants of obesity. *Healthlink. The Health Promotion Journal of the ACT Region,* 10-1.

Dunkley T.L., Wertheim E.H. & Paxton S.J. (2001). Examination of a model of multiple sociocultural influences on adolescent girls' body dissatisfaction and dietary restraint. *Adolescence 36*(142), 65–279.

Franklin, J., Denyer, G., Steinbeck, K.S., Caterson, I.D. & Hill, A.J. (2006). Obesity and Risk of Low Self-esteem: A State-wide Survey of Australian Children. *Paediatrics, 118* (6), 2481–2487.

Field, A.E., Camargo, C.A., Taylor B.C., Berkey, C.S., Roberts, S.B. & Colditz, G.A. (2001). Peer, Parent, and Media Influences on the Development of Weight Concerns and Frequent Dieting among Preadolescent and Adolescent Girls and Boys. *Pediatrics, 107* (1), 54–60.

Find Thirty Every Day (2008). WA Department of Health.

Fisher, J.O. & Birch, L.L. (1999). Restricting access to foods and children's eating. *Appetite, 32,* 405–419.

Fraser-Thomas, J. L. Cote, J. & Deakin, J. (2005). Youth sport programs: An avenue to foster positive youth development. *Physical Education and Sport Pedagogy, 10* (1), 19–40.

Fredricks, J.A., Eccles, J.S. (2004). Parental influence on youth involvement in sports. In M.R. Weiss (ed.), *Developmental Sport and Exercise Psychology: A Lifespan Perspective,* pp.145–164. Morgantown, WV: Fitness Information Technology Inc.

Goodman S., Lewis P.R., Dixon A.J. & Travers C.A. (2002). Childhood obesity: Of growing urgency. *Medical Journal of Australia 176*(8):400–1.

Grogan, S. (2006). Body image and health: Contemporary perspectives. *Journal of Health Psychology,* 11 (4), 523–530.

Hands, B., Parker, H., Glasson, C. (2004). *Physical activity and nutrition levels in Western Australian schoolchildren and adolescents: Report.* Perth, Western Australia, Western Australian Government.

Holt, K.E. & Ricciardelli, L. A. (2008). Weight concerns among elementary school children: A review of prevention programs, *Body Image,* 5 (3), 233–243.

Jones, D.C. & Crawford, J.K. (2006). The peer appearance culture during adolescence: Gender and body mass variations. *Journal of Youth and Adolescence, 2,* 257–269.

Keery, K, B, Van den Berg, P. & Thompson, J.K. (2005). The impact of appearance-related teasing by family members, *Journal of Adolescent Health 3,* 120–127.

Kotler, P. & Roberto, E. (1989). Social marketing: Strategies changing public health behaviour. In *Charter for Active Kids. A blueprint for active and healthy children in Western Australia.* Children's Physical Activity Coalition.

Littleton, H. L. & Ollendick, T. (2003). Negative Body Image and Disordered Eating Behavior in Children and Adolescents: What Places Youth at Risk and How Can These Problems Be Prevented? *Clinical Child & Family Psychology Review,* 6 (1), 51–66.

Magarey A.M., Daniels, L.A. & Boulton, T.J.C. (2001). Prevalence of overweight and   obesity in Australian children and adolescents: Reassessment of 1985 and 1995 data against new standard international definitions. *Medical Journal of Australia, 174*:561–4.

Marston, A.R., Jacobs, D.F., Singer, R.D., Widaman, K.F. & Little, T.D. (1988). Adolescents who apparently are invulnerable to drug, alcohol, and nicotine use. *Adolescence. 23*(91):593–8.

Malina, R.M. (1996). Tracking of physical activity and physical fitness across the lifespan. *Research Quarterly for Exercise and Sport, 67* (3), 548–557.

McCabe, M., Ricciardelli, L., Stanford, J., Holt, K., Keegan, S. & Miller, L. (2007). Where is all the pressure coming from? Messages from mothers and teachers about preschool children's appearance, diet and exercise, *European Eating Disorders Review*, vol. 15, no. 3, pp. 221–230.

McCabe, M., Ricciardelli, L. & Salmon, J. (2006). Evaluation of a prevention program to address body focus and negative affect among children, *Journal of Health Psychology*, 11 (4), 589–598.

McCabe, M. & Ricciardelli, L. (2005). A prospective study of pressures from parents, peers, and the media on extreme weight change behaviours among adolescent boys and girls, *Behaviour Research and Therapy*, 43 (5), 653–668.

McCabe, M., Ricciardelli, L., Mellor, D. & Ball, K. (2005). Media influences on body image and disordered eating among Indigenous adolescent Australians, *Adolescence*, 40 (157), 115–127.

Mellor, D, Fuller-Tyszkiewicz, M, McCabe, M .P. & Ricciardelli, L A. (2010). Body image and self-esteem across age and gender: A short-term longitudinal study, *Sex roles*, 1–10.

Mitchie, S., Abraham, C., Whittington, C., McAteer, J., Gupta, S. (2009). Effective Techniques in Healthy Eating and Physical Activity Interventions: A Meta-Regression. *Health Psychology, 28* (6), 690–701.

Myles, F.S., Scanlon, K.S., Birch, L.L., Francis, L.A. &http://www.nature.com/oby/journal/v12/n11/abs/oby2004212a.html - aff3 Sherry, B. (2004). Parent–Child Feeding Strategies and Their Relationships to Child Eating and Weight Status. *Obesity Research*) 12, 1711–1722.

National Eating Disorders Collaboration (2009). Funded by the Federal Department of Health and Ageing. *An evidence based National Framework on the prevention, treatment and management of eating disorders in Australia.* Butterfly Foundation.

National Health Priority Action Council (2006). *National Chronic Disease Strategy,* Australian Government Department of Health and Aging, Canberra.

National Obesity Taskforce (2003). *Healthy Weight 2008 — Australia's future. The national action agenda for children and young people and their families.*

National Obesity Task Force (2003). *Healthy Weight 2008 — Australia's Future.* Department of Health & Ageing: Canberra.

O'Dea, J. (2004). Evidence for a self-esteem approach in the prevention of body image and eating problems among children and adolescents. *Eating Disorders, 12,* 225–239.

O'Dea, J.A. (2007). Everybody's different: A positive approach to teaching about health, puberty, body image, nutrition, self-esteem and obesity prevention. Camberwell: ACER Press.

O'Dea, J.A. & Abraham, S. (2000). Improving the body image, eating attitudes, and behaviors of young male and female adolescents: A new educational approach that focuses on self-esteem. *International Journal of Eating Disorders, 28,* 43–57.

Owen, N., Bauman, A., Booth, M. (1995). Serial mass-media campaigns to promote physical activity: Reinforcing or redundant? *American Journal of Public Health, 85* (2), 244–248.

Pate, R.R., Baranowski, T., Dowda, M. & Trost, S.G. (1996). Tracking of physical activity in young children. *Medicine and Science in Exercise and Sports, 28,* 92–96.

Paxton, S., Eisenberg, M., Neumark-Sztiner, D. (2006). Prospective predictors of body dissatisfaction in adolescent girls and boys: A five-year longitudinal study. *Developmental Psychology, 42* (5), 888–899.

Piggford, M. Raciti, M., Harker, D. & Harker, M. (2008). Young adults' food motives. An Australian social marketing perspective, *Young Consumers: Insight and Ideas for Responsible Marketers, 9,* 17–28.

Puhl, R.M. & Latner, J.D. (2007). Stigma, obesity, and the health of the nation's children. *Psychological Bulletin, 133*(4), 557–580.

Poutanen, R, Lahti, S., Tolvanen, M. & Hausen, H. (2007). Gender differences in child-related and parent-related determinants of oral health-related lifestyle among 11- to 12-year-old Finnish schoolchildren. *Acta Odontologica Scandinavica, 65* (4), 194–200.

Rangan, A.M., Randall, D, Hector, D.J., Gill, T.P. & Webb, K.L. (2008). Consumption of 'extra' foods by Australian children: Types, quantities and contribution to energy and nutrient intakes. 'Extra' food consumption. *European Journal of Clinical Nutrition, 62,* 356–364

Ricciardeli, L. & McCabe, M. (2001). Children's body image concerns and eating disturbance: A review of the literature. *Clinical Psychology Review, 21* (3), 325–344.

Rich, E. & Evans, J. (2008). Learning to be healthy, dying to be thin: The representation of weight via body perfection codes in schools. In S. Riley, M. Burns, H. Frith, S. Wiggins & P. Markula (eds), Critical bodies: Representations, identities and practices of weight and body management, pp. 60–76. London: Palgrave/McMillan.

Scaglioni, S., Salvioni, M. & Galimberti, C. (2008). Influence of parental attitudes in the development of children's eating behaviour. *British Journal of Nutrition, 99* (1), 122–125.

Schur, E., Sanders, M. & Steiner, H. (2000). Body dissatisfaction and dieting in young children. *International Journal of Eating Disorders, 27,* 74–82.

Smolak, L. (2004). Body image in children and adolescents: Where do we go from here? *Body Image, 1,* 15–28.

Smolak, L., Levine, M.P. & Schermer, F. (1999). Parental input in weight concerns among elementary school children. *International Journal of Eating Disorders, 25,* 263–272.

Tennant S., Hetzel D. & Glover J. (2003). *A social health atlas of young South Australians*, 2nd edn. Adelaide: Openbook Print.

Vaska V.L. & Volkmer R. (2004). Increasing prevalence of obesity in South Australian 4-year-olds: 1995–2002. *Journal of Paediatric Child Health, 40,* 353–5.

Wertheim, E.H., Mee, V. & Paxton, S.J. (1999). Relationships among adolescent girls' eating behaviours and their parents' weight related attitudes and behaviors. *Sex Roles, 41,* 169–187.

World Health Organization (2000). *Obesity: Preventing and managing the global epidemic.* Report of a WHO consultation.

World Health Organization (2003). *Diet, nutrition and the prevention of chronic diseases.* World Health Organization.

Appendices

Goal setting help sheet

What are my SMART goals? Specific, Measurable, Achievable, Realistic, Time. (Come up with as many as you'd like).

What specific, realistic and achievable changes do I want to see in my *attitude*?

How will I measure its achievement?

What's the time frame for achievement?

What specific, realistic and achievable changes do I want to see in my *behaviour*?

How will I measure its achievement?

What's the time frame for achievement?

What changes do I want to see in my *thinking*? What are my SMART goals?

How will I measure this change?

What's the time frame?

Erasing rituals and facing fears
Erasing ritualistic behaviour help sheet

Rituals I want to stop:

What are the benefits to stopping this ritual?

What are the steps to stopping this behaviour?

What strategies will I use to reduce my anxiety whilst trying to stop this ritual?

What reward will I give myself for stopping this ritual?

Developing fear hierarchy help sheet

What situations do I fear? Start with the biggest and work down to smallest. Rate out of 10 how much fear you feel thinking about being in this situation

1. (my biggest fear)

2.

3.

4.

5.

Developing fear hierarchy help sheet (continued)

6.

7.

8.

9.

10. (my smallest fear)

What are the steps leading up to facing and mastering this fear?

What can I do to reduce the fear? What relaxation etc. can I do?

How often will I need to practice facing the smaller fear before I move on to the next one?

What can I tell myself and think to reduce the fear? What coping statements will I tell myself?

What reward will I give myself for facing this fear?

What's the next step?

Basic and higher needs help sheet

What do I do that meets my *physical* needs?

What can I add to further meet these needs?

My SMART goal:

What do I do that meets my *spiritual* needs?

What can I add to further meet these needs?

My SMART goal:

What do I do that meets my *emotional* needs?

What can I add to further meet these needs?

My SMART goal:

What can I add to further meet my *career* needs?

What can I add to further meet these needs?

My SMART goal:

What can I add to further meet my *intellectual* needs?

What can I add to further meet these needs?

My SMART goal:

Services in Australia and Around the Globe
Where to get additional help

Australian Capital Territory

Eating Disorders Program
About: A specialist, community-based, multidisciplinary team providing assessment and treatment programs for people with eating disorders. Team includes: psychiatrist, psychologists and allied health professionals. Outpatient and day programs are available to residents of both the ACT and surrounding NSW regions. Consultation/liaison is also available to health professionals.
Address: Phillip Health Centre, Cnr Keltie and Corinna Streets, Woden, ACT 2606
Telephone: (02) 6205 1519
Fax: (02) 6205 1152
1 800 621 354 for 24 hours Crisis Team

Mental Illness ACT
About: MIEACT educates the Canberra community about mental illness. It aims to reduce stigma and discrimination, improve knowledge, and to raise awareness about the importance of getting help early.
Website: www.mieact.org.au/

Victoria

Eating Disorders Foundation of Victoria
About: A non-profit organisation which supports those affected by eating disorders and aims to better inform the community about disordered eating.

Address: 1513 High Street, Glen Iris,Vic 3146
   Telephone: (03) 9885 0318
   Fax: (03) 9885 1153
   Non-metro Victorian callers call 1300 550 236
   (helpline)
   Website: www.eatingdisorders.org.au
   Email: edfv@eatingdisorders.org.au

New South Wales

The Butterfly Foundation
About: The Butterfly Foundation is dedicated to bring change to
culture, policy and practice in the prevention, treatment and
support of those affected by eating disorders and negative body
image. It has a telephone helpline for people with eating disorders
and their family and friends. Support is also available via email.
Address: 103 Alexander Street, Crows Nest, NSW 2065
   Telephone: 1800 33 4673
   Fax: 02 8090 8196
   Website: www.thebutterflyfoundation.org.au
   Email: support@thebutterflyfoundation.org.au

Queensland

Eating Disorders Association Inc. Queensland
About: A non-profit organisation that provides information,
support and referral services.
Address: 12 Chatsworth Road, Greenslopes, Qld 4120
   Telephone: (07) 3394 3661
   Fax: (07) 3394 3663
   Website: www.eda.org.au
   Email: admin@eda.org.au

South Australia

Aceda

About: A not for profit community organisation to support people with eating disorders.

Address: Everard House, 589 South Road, Everard Park, SA 5035

Telephone: (08) 8297 4088

Fax: (08) 8297 7587

Website: www.aceda.org.au

Email: aceda@aceda.org.au

Western Australia

Women's Health Works

About: A non-profit community organisation that provides a range of education, information and support services to women, including self-help groups for people experiencing an eating disorder.

Address: Suite 6, Joondalup Lotteries House, 70 Davidson Tce, Joondalup, WA 6919

Telephone: (08) 9300 1566

Fax: (08) 9300 1699

Website: www.womenshealthworks.org.au

Email: info@womenshealthworks.org.au

ARAFMI Mental Health Carers & Friends Association Inc.

About: A non-profit community based organisation that provides information and support for families and friends of people with

mental health issues, including: family support counselling, support group program advocacy, respite and community education.
Address: 182–188 Lord Street, Perth, WA 6000
Telephone: (08) 9427 7100 or
1800 811 747 (rural freecall)
Fax: (08) 9427 7119
Website: www.arafmi.asn.au

Centre for Clinical Intervention (CCI)
About: A free, specialist, state-wide mental health program offering cognitive behavioural therapy for people with eating disorders, as well as other mental health conditions.
Address: 223 James Street, Northbridge, WA 6003
Telephone: (08) 9227 6003
Fax: (08) 9328 5911
Website: www.cci.health.wa.gov.au
Email: info.cci@health.wa.gov.au

Tasmania

Tasmanian Eating Disorders Website
About: This site provides online information and resources for people with eating disorders and support groups for sufferers and carers.
Contact: Telephone: (03) 6222 7222
Website: www.tas.eatingdisorders.org.au
Email: tas.eatingdisorders@dhhs.tas.gov.au

Across Australia

Australian Psychological Society
About: The professional association of psychologists. For referral to a psychologist in your area. Also, to access tip-sheets and infor-

mation on evidence-based therapy and assistance in Australia. Tip sheet on Eating disorders and link to assistance:
http://www.psychology.org.au/community/eating_disorders/
Website: www.psychology.org.au

Headspace

About: Provides young people aged 12–25 years and their families with information, support and advice on general health, mental health and wellbeing, alcohol and other drugs, education, employment and other services. There are several locations across Australia.
Website: www.headspace.org.au

Nutrition Society of Australia

For information on nutrition and services in Australia.
Website: www.nsa.asn.au

Nutrition Australia

For information on nutrition and services in Australia
Website: www.nutritionaustralia.org

Dieticians Association of Australia

For referrals to a nutritionist or dietician
Website: daa.asn.au

New Zealand

Eating Difficulties Education Network (EDEN)

About: A non-profit community agency based in Auckland, Aotearoa New Zealand.

Address:1 Garnet Road, Westmere, Auckland, New Zealand
　　　　Telephone: (09) 378 9039
　　　　Fax: (09) 378 9393
　　　　Website: www.eden.org.nz
　　　　Email: info@eden.org.nz

United Kindom

British Psychological Society

About: The professional association of psychologists. For referral to a psychologist. Also, to access tip-sheets and information on evidence-based therapy and assistance in the UK.
Website: www.bps.org.uk

The Centre for Appearance Research

About: The Centre for Appearance Research (CAR) coducts research and assists people living with appearance related concerns. It is part of the University of the West of England.
Website: www1.uwe.ac.uk/hls/research/appearanceresearch

United States

National Eating Disorders Association

About: It supports individuals and families affected by eating disorders.
Website: www.nationaleatingdisorders.org

New Zealand

Eating Difficulties Education Network (EDEN)
About: A non-profit community agency based in Auckland, Aotearoa New Zealand.
Address:1 Garnet Road, Westmere, Auckland, New Zealand
Telephone: (09) 378 9039
Fax: (09) 378 9393
Website: www.eden.org.nz
Email: info@eden.org.nz

United Kingdom

British Psychological Society
About: The professional association of psychologists. For referral to a psychologist. Also, to access tip-sheets and information on evidence-based therapy and assistance in the UK.
Website: www.bps.org.uk

The Centre for Appearance Research
About: The Centre for Appearance Research (CAR) conducts research and assist people living with appearance related concerns. It is part of the University of the West of England.
Website: www1.uwe.ac.uk/hls/research/appearanceresearch

United States

National Eating Disorders Association
About: It supports individuals and families affected by eating disorders.
Website: www.nationaleatingdisorders.org

www.ingramcontent.com/pod-product-compliance
Lightning Source LLC
Chambersburg PA
CBHW061731270326
41928CB00011B/2198